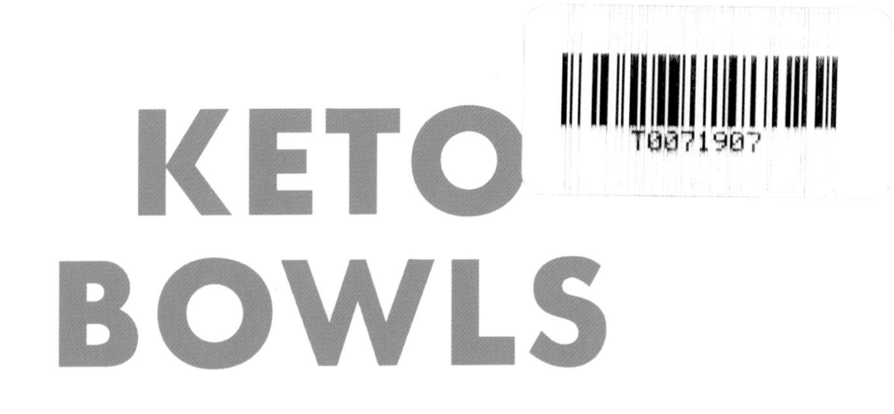

KETO BOWLS

KETO BOWLS

SIMPLE AND DELICIOUS LOW-CARB, HIGH-FAT RECIPES FOR YOUR KETOGENIC LIFESTYLE

PAMELA ELLGEN

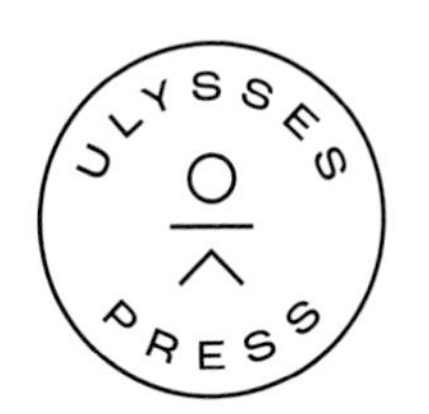

Published in the U.S. by:
ULYSSES PRESS
P.O. Box 3440
Berkeley, CA 94703
www.ulyssespress.com

ISBN: 978-1-64604-001-8
Library of Congress Control Number: 2019951344

Printed in the United States by Versa Press
10 9 8 7 6 5 4 3 2 1

Acquisitions editor: Bridget Thoreson
Managing editor: Claire Chun
Project editor: Renee Rutledge
Editor: Miriam Jones
Proofreader: Ruby Privateer
Cover design: Rebecca Lown
Cover photographs: Pamela Ellgen

NOTE TO READERS: This book has been written and published strictly for informational and educational purposes only. It is not intended to serve as medical advice or to be any form of medical treatment. You should always consult your physician before altering or changing any aspect of your medical treatment and/or undertaking a diet regimen, including the guidelines as described in this book. Do not stop or change any prescription medications without the guidance and advice of your physician. Any use of the information in this book is made on the reader's good judgment after consulting with his or her physician and is the reader's sole responsibility. This book is not intended to diagnose or treat any medical condition and is not a substitute for a physician.

This book is independently authored and published and no sponsorship or endorsement of this book by, and no affiliation with, any trademarked brands or other products mentioned within is claimed or suggested. All trademarks that appear in ingredient lists and elsewhere in this book belong to their respective owners and are used here for informational purposes only. The author and publisher encourage readers to patronize the quality brands mentioned and pictured in this book.

CONTENTS

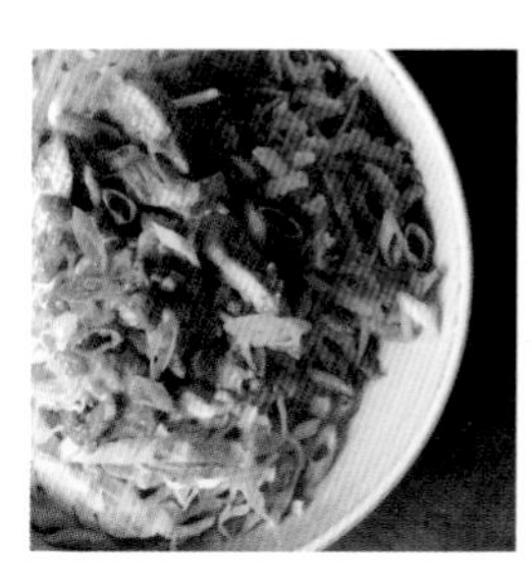

CHAPTER THREE

CHICKEN. 26

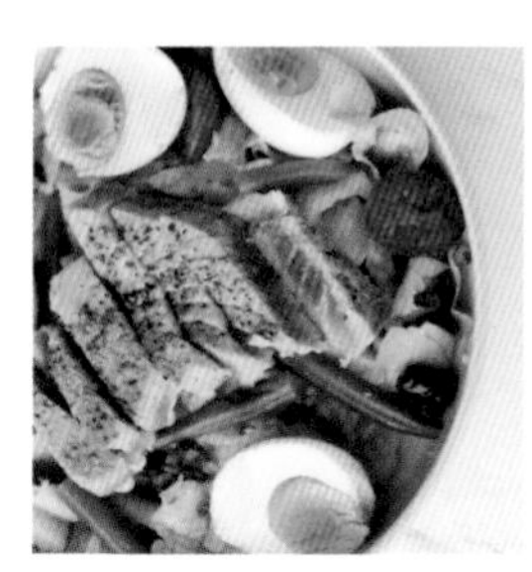

CHAPTER FOUR

FISH & SEAFOOD 40

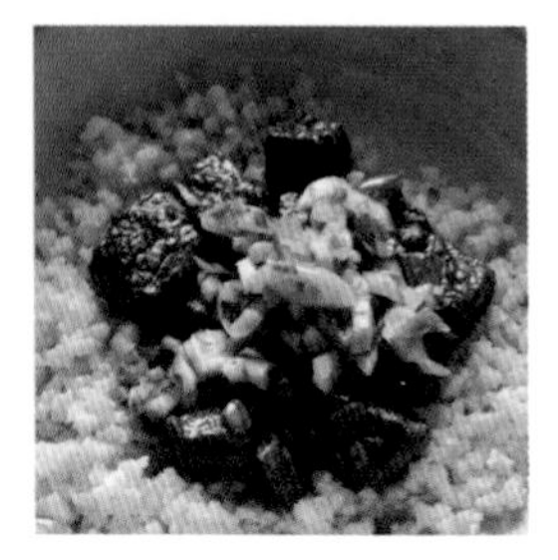

CHAPTER FIVE

BEEF & LAMB 54

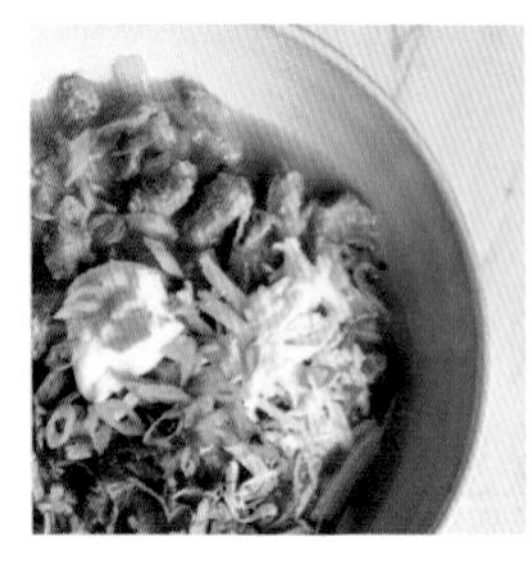

CHAPTER SIX

PORK 72

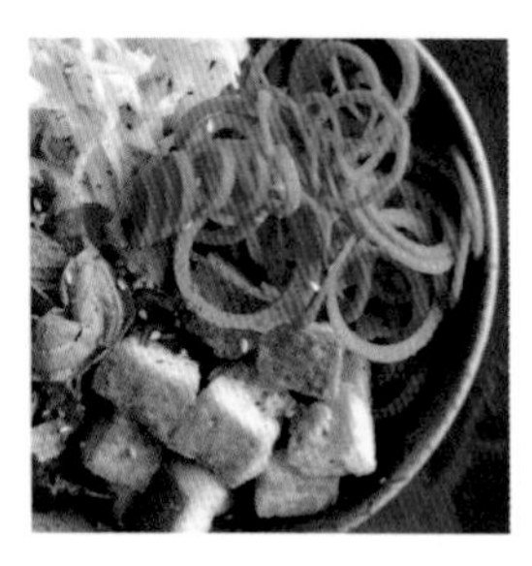

CHAPTER SEVEN

VEGETARIAN 84

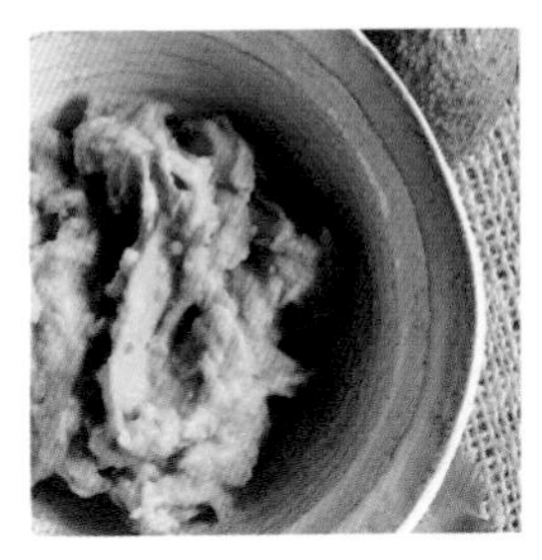

CHAPTER EIGHT

BASICS 96

INTRODUCTION

Do you look longingly at the brightly colored bowl meals that fill your Pinterest feed? They're a one-dish feast for the eyes. They're also loaded with carbs—heaps of rice topped with loads of legumes topped with sweetened dried fruit and drowning in a sticky sweet dressing. Oh my!

Keto Bowls offers a low-carb alternative to these carb bombs. You don't need to stray from your keto diet to enjoy bright, colorful bowl meals. It just takes a few simple swaps—and don't worry, that's not code for "just replace it with meat."

From breakfast to dinner, the Keto Bowls Cookbook invites you to craft tasty bowls with low-carb foods. For breakfast, try the Cashew Yogurt Bowl with Toasted Coconut and Almond Butter, salty sweet Nut and Seed Granola with Olive Oil (for real, it's delicious!), or Smoked Salmon and Spinach Scramble.

For lunch, try the classic Niçoise Salad Bowl, Green Goddess Chicken with Jicama Noodles, or Curried Cauliflower and Tofu Bowls with Arugula. For dinner, try the Roasted Chicken bowls or the comforting Meatballs over Mashed Cauliflower.

There is also a vegetarian chapter for those days when you simply need a break from animal foods or you want to lighten your carbon footprint while staying keto. Try the Vibrant Tofu Carrot Noodle Bowl.

If you're new to keto, the basics chapter will be your best friend. It offers those recipes that everyone else seems to already know how to make but may be somewhat intimidating your first time, including cauliflower rice, spaghetti squash, spiralized vegetables, and a versatile creamy herb vinaigrette.

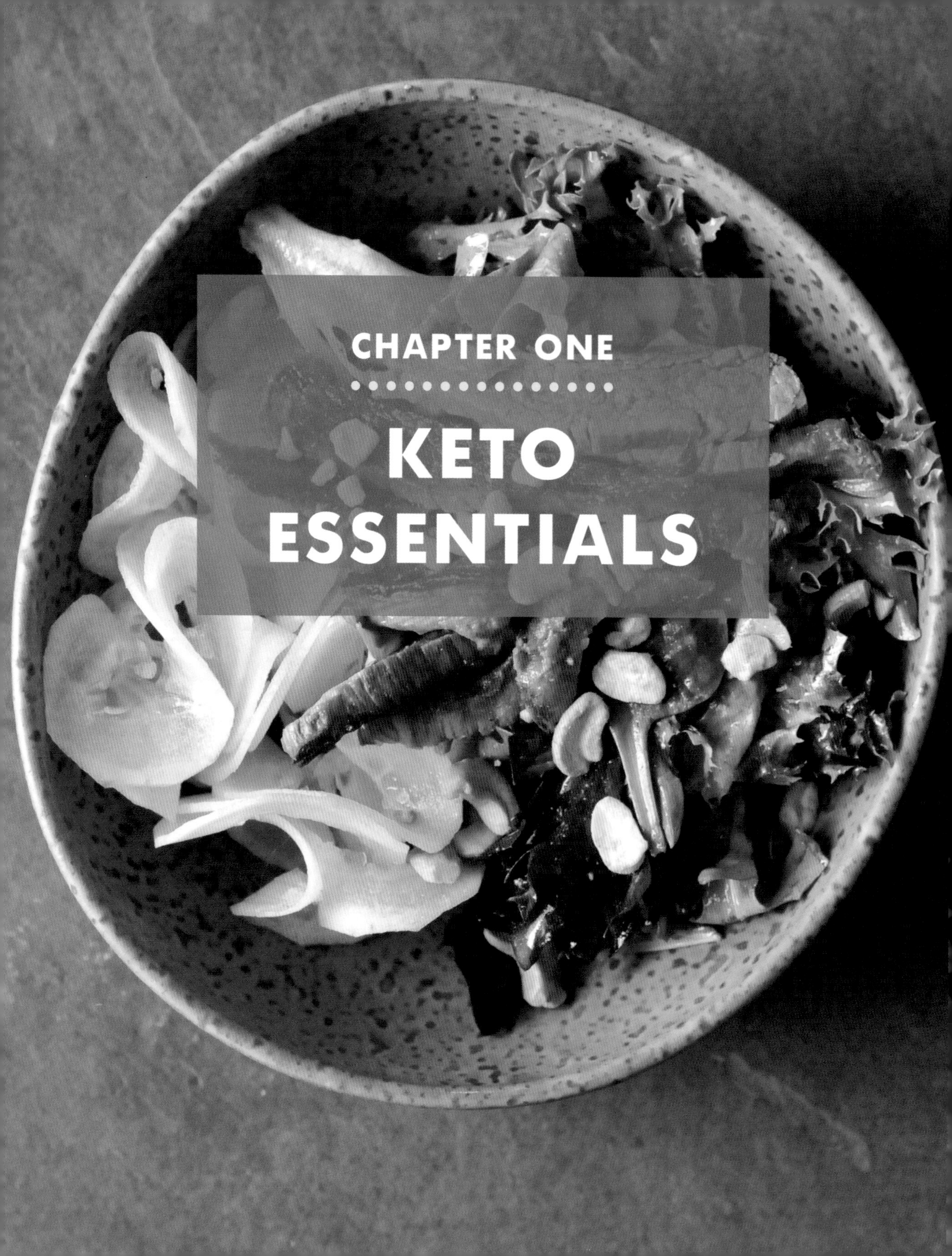

CHAPTER ONE

KETO ESSENTIALS

Whether you come to the ketogenic diet to lose weight, improve mental clarity, or heal chronic health conditions, you want delicious low-carb meals that keep you in ketosis. That can easily translate into a steady diet of bacon and eggs for breakfast, avocado and chicken thighs for lunch, and steak and asparagus topped with butter for dinner. Boring. While these might technically keep you keto, they're not very fun—or healthy long term.

Go to a keto cookbook for inspiration and you might find, as I did, that many begin with the premise that you want to recreate all of the junk foods you enjoyed on a Standard American Diet but with low-carb foods. Pork dust tortillas, anyone?

Not in my book.

The idea behind bowl meals is that you can get all of the nutrients you need in a simple, colorful bowl. It's designed to be healthy—we're not trying to recreate cheesecake here—but it usually means lots of carbs.

In this book, recipes are built around non-starchy vegetables for volume and whole-food fat and protein sources for calories. My goal is to replace grains and legumes that form the basis of most bowl meals with low-carb alternatives—replacing brown rice, whole-grain pasta, and grain-based granola with riced cauliflower, zucchini noodles, and nut and seed granola, respectively.

WHAT IS KETO?

The bare-bones keto diet involves a diet composed of 70 percent (or more) fat, 20 percent protein, and 5 to 10 percent carbohydrate. If you're eating roughly 1,800 calories a day, that breaks down to 140 grams of fat, 90 grams of protein, and 22 to 45 grams of carbohydrate. Many people on keto opt for even fewer grams of total carbs. Ultimately, do what works for your body and helps you achieve your health goals.

The types of carbs matter on a keto diet—you can't just go eat a bag or two of potato chips and call that your carb allotment. Where they come from, how processed they are, and how much fiber they contain matters. In this book, the primary sources of carbs are vegetables, nuts and seeds, and to a very limited extent, low-sugar fruit such as berries. You may notice the recipes in this book have a few more total carbs than many keto recipes. One reason is that this book incorporates more whole plant foods, which are essential to your health on or off a keto diet. Look at net carbs for the actual carb value.

Protein is also a hot topic on keto. Too much can send you straight out of keto because your body can use it to make glucose. So, you can't just load up on muscle meat (thank goodness) and call it keto. It doesn't work that way.

The keto diet bears many similarities to paleo, primal, and Whole30 approaches to food. So, if you're also following one of those diets, you'll find many of the recipes in this book compatible. A few key differences are that some recipes call for nonnutritive sweeteners, peanut butter, and dairy. Additionally, those diets are less concerned with macros than keto is. However, I am sensitive to the fact that many people can't do dairy, whether due to lactose intolerance or an outright allergy. Hence, many of the recipes in this book are also dairy-free.

There are many books written on the science behind keto. This isn't one of them. I've provided several in the references section for you to check out.

WHAT TO EAT

The essential ingredients in a keto diet come straight from the earth and bring so much flavor to your plate—vibrant vegetables, hearty nuts and seeds, savory meats, fresh seafood, and creamy dairy and eggs. Oils, vinegars, herbs, spices, and even some low-sugar fruits keep it interesting.

Vegetables

- bell peppers
- bok choy
- broccoli
- brussels sprouts
- cabbage
- cauliflower
- celery
- cucumber
- eggplant
- fennel
- garlic
- herbs
- kale
- leafy greens
- mushrooms
- onions
- spaghetti squash
- spinach
- tomatoes
- zucchini

Fruits

Choose low-carb fruits like berries and citrus.

- avocado
- blueberries
- grapefruit
- lemons

- limes
- oranges
- raspberries
- strawberries

Meat and Fish

- beef
- chicken
- duck
- fish
- lamb
- pork
- shellfish
- turkey
- wild game

Nuts and Seeds

- almonds
- cashews
- hazelnuts
- macadamia nuts
- peanuts (technically a legume)
- pecans
- pine nuts
- pistachios
- sesame seeds
- walnuts

Dairy and Eggs

- butter
- cheese
- eggs
- heavy cream
- yogurt, full-fat (dairy and plant-based)

Oils

- coconut oil
- ghee
- olive oil

Sweeteners

- erythritol
- monk fruit
- stevia (limit)

Other Foods

- almond flour
- bone broth
- coconut flour
- dark chocolate
- herbs and spices
- mayonnaise
- mustard
- red wine
- vinegars

WHAT TO AVOID

Starchy Vegetables

Not all vegetables are created equal. Stay away from starchy choices such as:

- acorn squash
- butternut squash
- corn
- kabocha squash
- potatoes
- pumpkin
- sweet potatoes
- winter squashes
- yams
- yucca

High-Carb Fruits

- apples
- bananas
- dried fruit
- grapes
- peaches
- plantains

Grains and Grain Products

- bread
- oats
- pasta
- pastries
- quinoa (technically a seed)
- rice

Legumes

- beans
- chickpeas
- lentils
- peas

Low-Fat/Non-Fat Dairy

- low-fat cheeses
- low-fat milk
- low-fat yogurt

Sweeteners

- agave
- high-fructose corn syrup
- honey
- maple syrup
- molasses
- sugar

Other Foods

- beer
- candy
- chips
- crackers
- "nutrition" bars
- processed foods

HELPFUL TOOLS

Here are the essential pieces of equipment in my kitchen:

Blender: A blender is helpful for pureeing sauces and soups. Either a countertop or immersion blender will work.

Food processor: A food processor can help make sauces such as pesto and prepare riced cauliflower. However, a sharp chef's knife and a box grater work equally well if you're willing to spend a few extra minutes chopping and grating.

Sheet pan: A rimmed baking sheet is great for roasting vegetables and meats. Because of its low sides, it helps with browning but keeps foods and liquids from spilling.

Skillet: One large (12 to 14 inches) and one small (10 inches).

Spiralizer: Vegetable noodles are the base for many recipes in this book, so invest in a simple countertop spiralizer. The handheld versions don't yield very good results.

***

Look for these recipe labels:

dairy free **DF** | gluten free **GF** | nut free **NF** | vegan **Vg** | vegetarian **V**

CHAPTER TWO

BREAKFAST

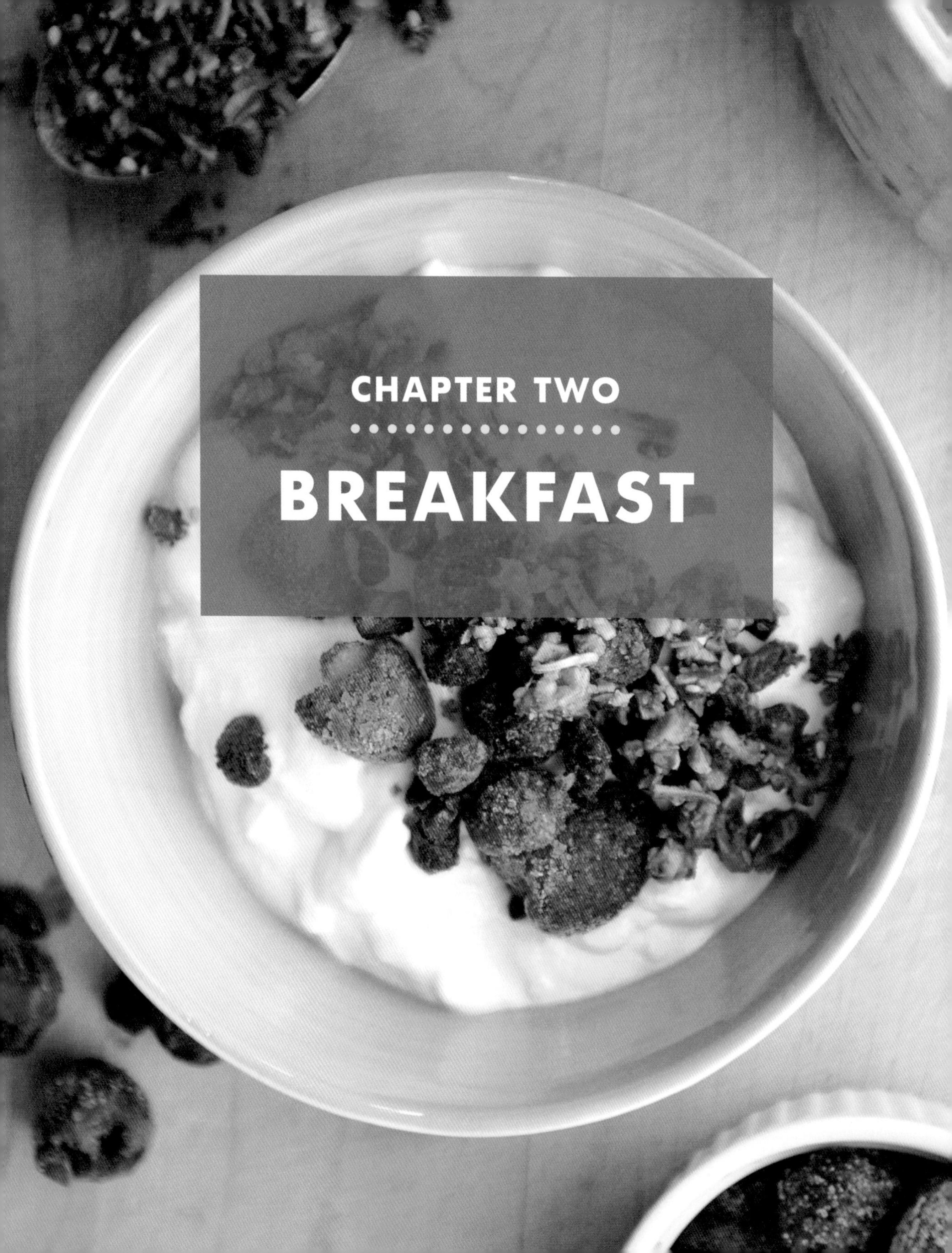

You may not need or want breakfast on a keto diet. Intermittent fasting—not eating for a period of time as short as a single meal or as long as a day or more—can improve metabolism, mental clarity, and weight loss. When you do eat breakfast, these tasty meals will keep you in ketosis and provide a delicious way to start your day.

- Açai Bowl with Pepitas, Coconut, and Chia
- Nut and Seed Granola with Olive Oil
- Berry Coconut Yogurt Bowl with Granola
- Cashew Yogurt Bowl with Toasted Coconut and Almond Butter
- Sunshine Ricotta Bowls with Granola
- Macadamia Coconut Porridge
- Rosemary Sautéed Mushrooms with Wilted Spinach and Scrambled Eggs
- BLT Scramble Bowl
- Roasted Vegetables and Sausage with Eggs and Sriracha
- Smoked Salmon and Spinach Scramble

Açai Bowls with Pepitas, Coconut, and Chia DF GF NF Vg

When açai bowls first flooded the streets of Los Angeles, I was working as a health editor for a website and couldn't believe how anyone could feel good after eating these carb bombs. Some bowls had as much sugar as a large soda. But, after interviewing a competitive surfer out of Hawaii who swore by them, I knew I had to give them a try, and of course put a low-carb spin on them.

YIELD: 2 servings | **PREP TIME:** 5 minutes | **COOK TIME:** 0 minutes

2 (100-gram) packs frozen açai puree

1 cup full-fat coconut milk

4 to 5 drops liquid stevia

2 tablespoons pepitas

2 tablespoons shredded unsweetened coconut

1 tablespoon chia seeds

1. Combine the frozen açai, coconut milk, and stevia in a blender. Puree until smooth.
2. Divide between serving bowls and top with the pepitas, coconut, and chia seeds.

NUTRITION PER SERVING

CALORIES: 382 TOTAL FAT: 33g PROTEIN: 11g CARBOHYDRATES: 11g FIBER: 7g NET CARBS: 4g

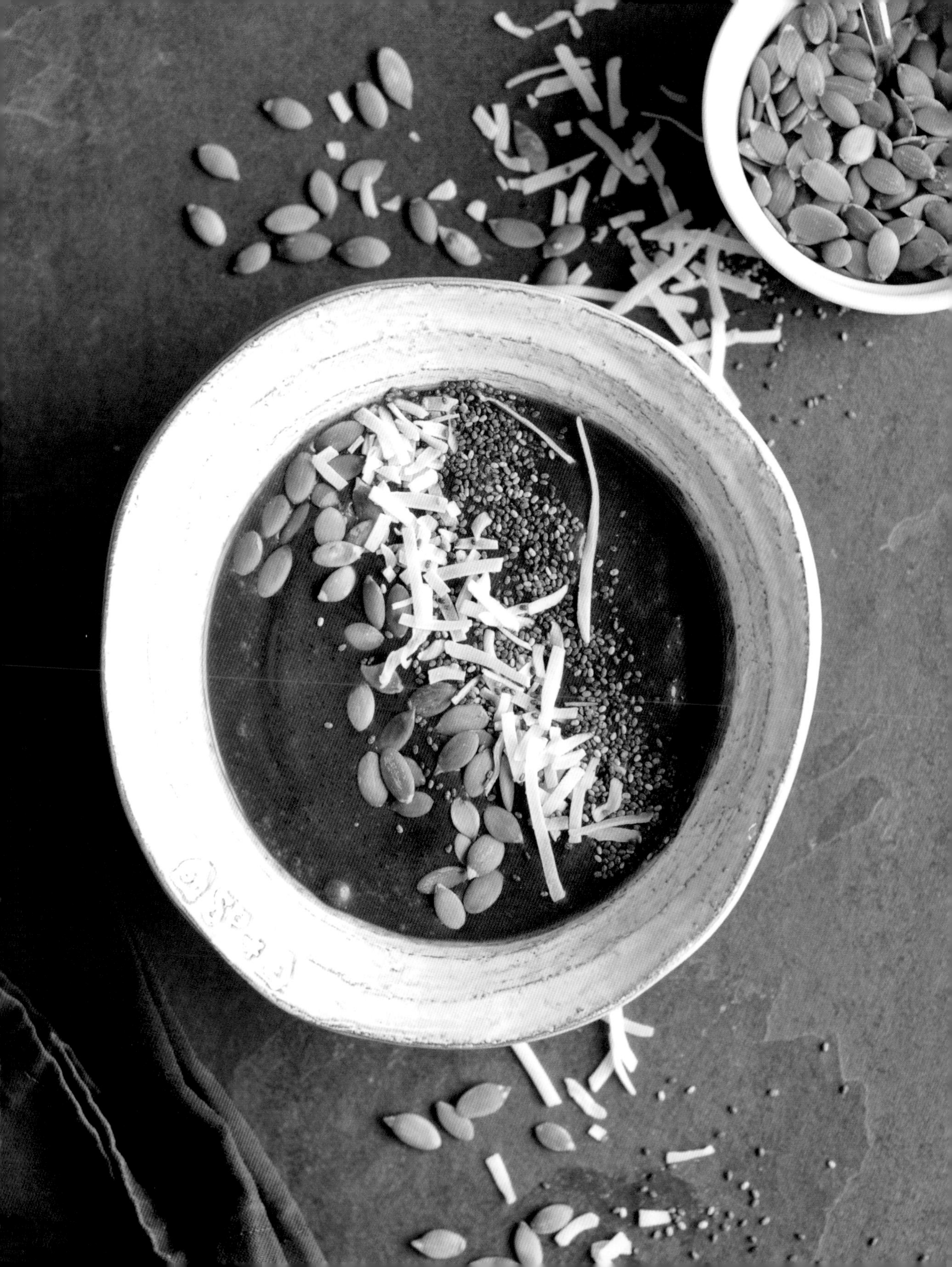

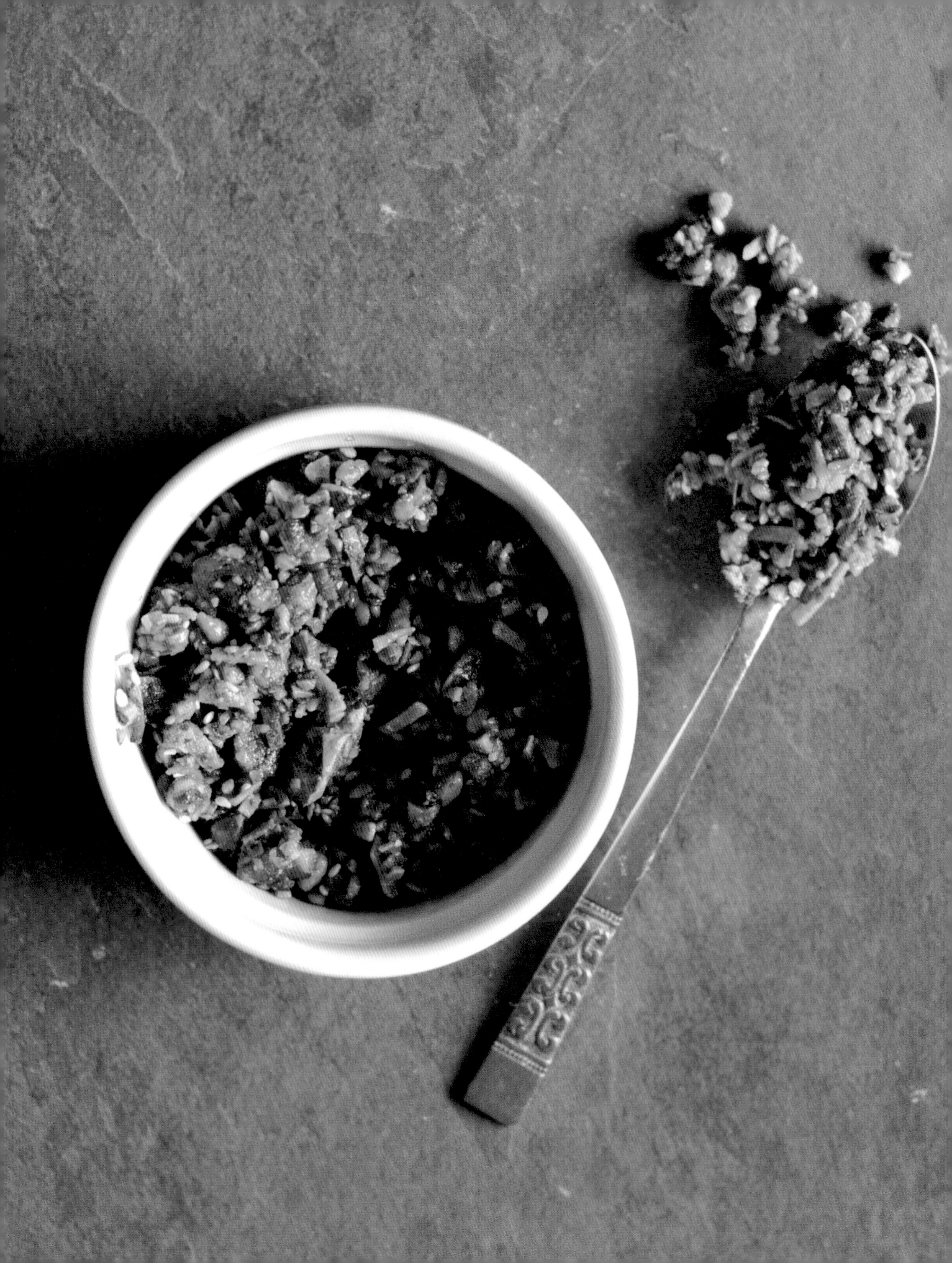

Nut and Seed Granola with Olive Oil DF GF Vg

I really prefer cold breakfast to something hot, rich, and savory. So, when I stopped eating granola, I knew I needed a replacement that satisfied my desire for something sweet and crunchy. This version is delicious sprinkled over yogurt or served with milk.

YIELD: 5 cups or 10 (½-cup) servings | **PREP TIME:** 5 minutes | **COOK TIME:** 40 minutes

- 2 cups walnuts
- 1 cup Brazil nuts
- ½ cup pepitas
- ¼ cup sesame seeds
- 1 cup shredded unsweetened coconut
- ½ cup extra-virgin olive oil
- ½ cup granulated lakanto monk fruit sweetener (not liquid)
- ½ teaspoon sea salt
- 1 teaspoon vanilla extract

1. Preheat the oven to 325°F.
2. Place the walnuts and Brazil nuts into a food processor and pulse until finely chopped, but not ground. Add the pepitas, sesame seeds, and coconut. Pulse once or twice just to mix.
3. In a separate container, combine the olive oil, monk fruit, sea salt, and vanilla. Pour this mixture into the food processor and pulse once or twice to mix.
4. Spread the nut mixture onto a rimmed baking sheet. Bake for 10 minutes, then stir. Bake for another 10 minutes, then stir. Turn off the heat but return the pan to the oven with the door slightly ajar to set for another 20 minutes. Remove the pan from the oven and allow to cool completely before storing for up to one month.

INGREDIENT TIP: If olive oil seems strange to you in a granola, I get it. But please give it a chance! Its slight acidity brightens the granola and balances the sea salt and sweet monk fruit.

NUTRITION PER SERVING

CALORIES: 439 TOTAL FAT: 45g PROTEIN: 9g CARBOHYDRATES: 8g FIBER: 4g NET CARBS: 4g

Berry Coconut Yogurt Bowl with Granola GF V

Once you make the Nut and Seed Granola with Olive Oil, you'll want to pour it over everything. Or, maybe it's just me. This recipe—if you can even call it a recipe—is a quick and classic breakfast option with a low-carb twist. If you prefer a dairy-free option, swap the yogurt for plain cashew- or coconut-based yogurt.

YIELD: 1 serving | **PREP TIME:** 5 minutes | **COOK TIME:** 0 minutes

¾ cup plain whole-milk yogurt

2 tablespoons frozen berries

¼ cup Nut and Seed Granola with Olive Oil (page 13)

Place the yogurt into a serving bowl and top with the frozen berries and granola. Serve immediately.

NUTRITION PER SERVING

CALORIES: 340 TOTAL FAT: 28g PROTEIN: 11g CARBOHYDRATES: 14g FIBER: 3g NET CARBS: 11g

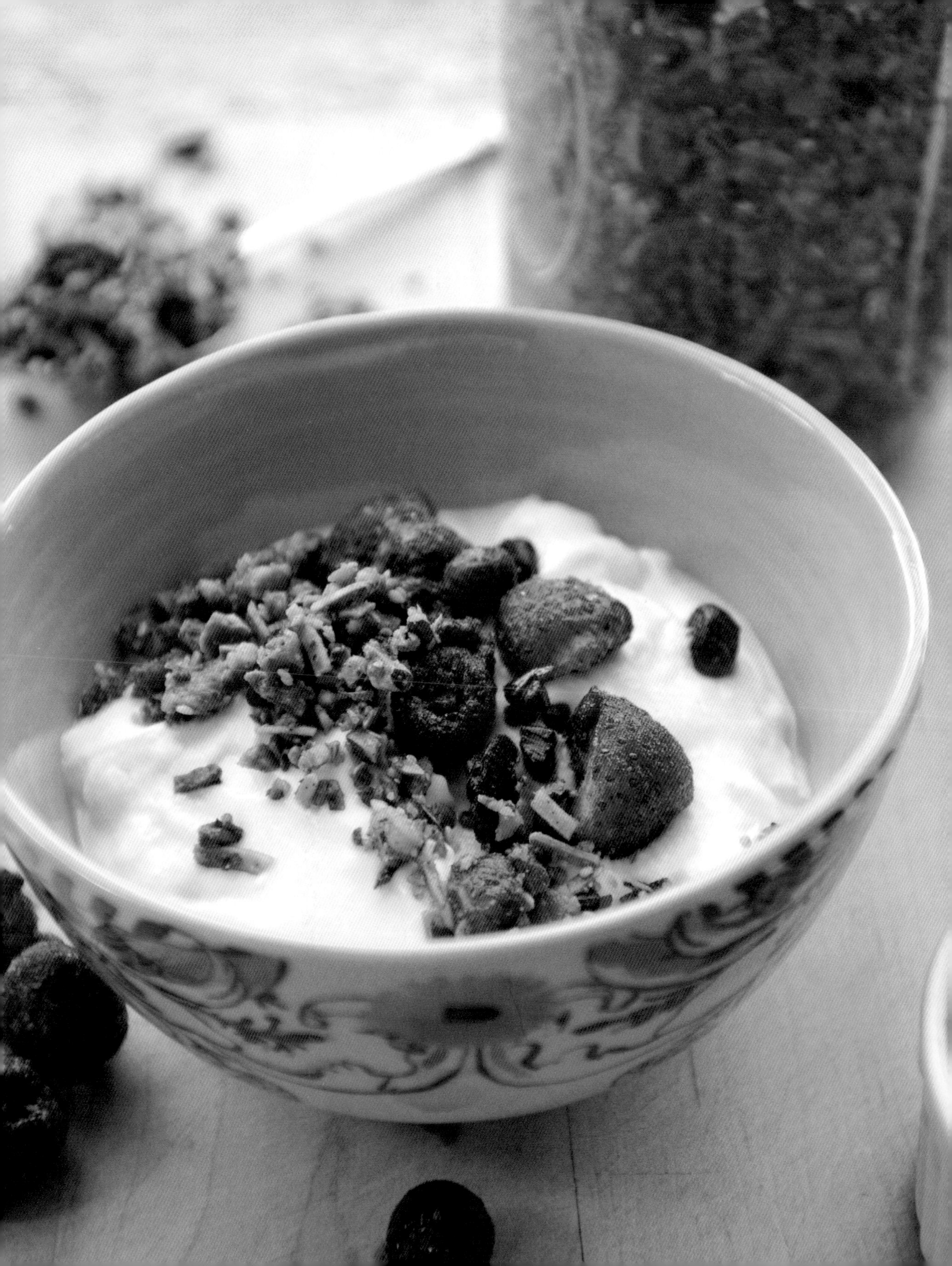

Cashew Yogurt Bowl with Toasted Coconut and Almond Butter DF GF Vg

This simple yogurt bowl drizzled with almond butter and toasted coconut is something I could eat every day. It's barely sweet and has all of the toasty flavors from the almond butter and coconut flakes. Add a couple tablespoons of blueberries for just two more grams of net carbs or leave them out if you want to save carbs for later in the day.

YIELD: 1 serving | **PREP TIME:** 5 minutes | **COOK TIME:** 0 minutes

1 cup plain full-fat cashew yogurt

1 tablespoon coconut oil, liquid

1 to 2 drops liquid stevia

1 tablespoon almond butter, warmed

2 tablespoons coconut flakes, toasted

2 tablespoons fresh or frozen blueberries (optional)

1. Place the cashew yogurt into a medium bowl and stir in the coconut oil and stevia.
2. Drizzle with the almond butter then top with the coconut flakes and blueberries, if using. Serve immediately.

INGREDIENT TIP: If you prefer to use a whole-milk yogurt in place of the cashew yogurt, that's fine. Just make sure whatever you use has no added sweeteners.

NUTRITION PER SERVING

CALORIES: 398 TOTAL FAT: 36g PROTEIN: 6g CARBOHYDRATES:17g FIBER: 4g NET CARBS: 13g

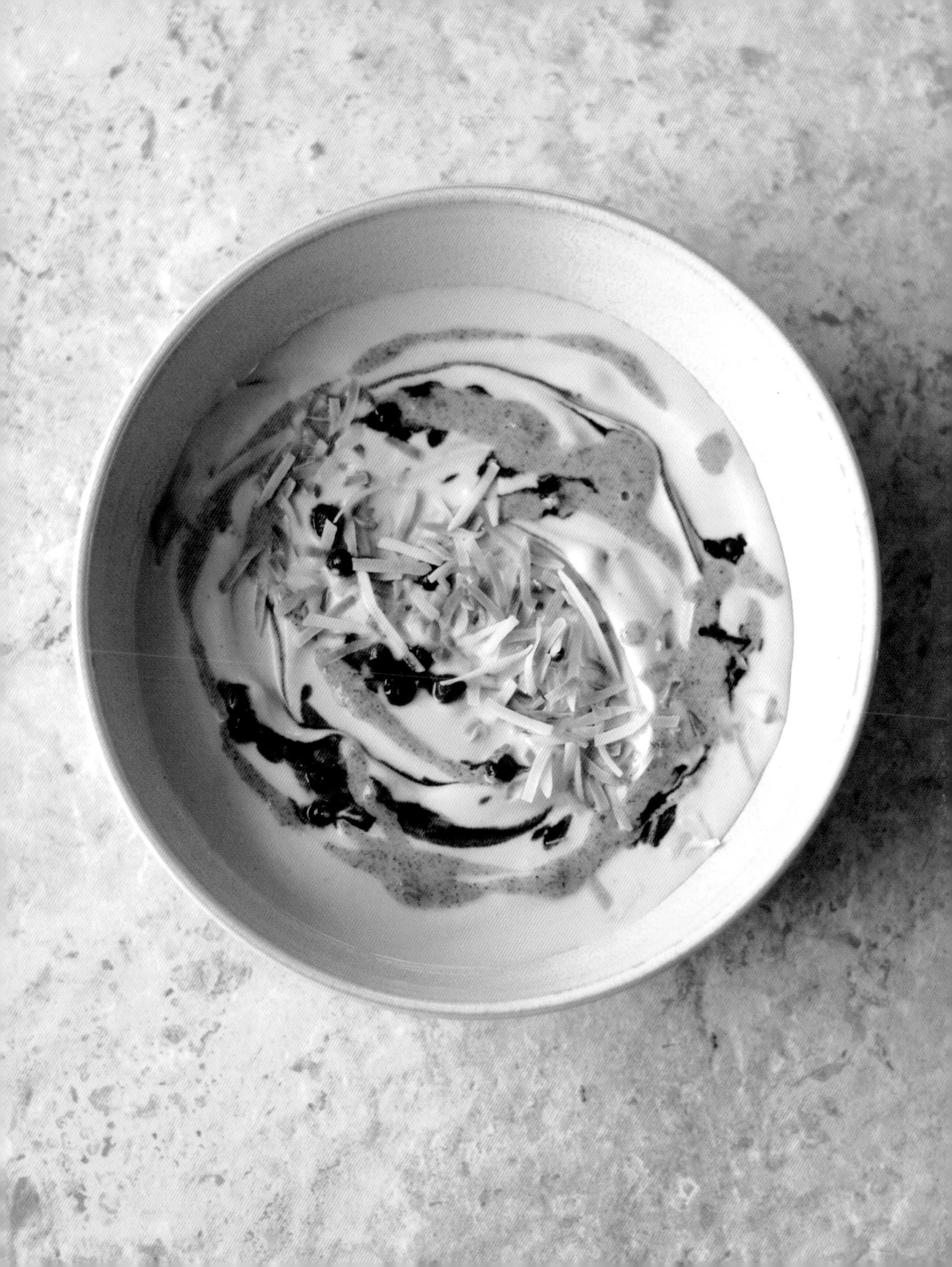

Sunshine Ricotta Bowls with Granola GF V

Brighten up your winter morning with these colorful ricotta bowls. The saltiness of the ricotta is a nice change of pace from yogurt—but feel free to swap it for a whole-milk yogurt if you prefer. The granola adds a nice crunch and flavor but can be replaced with a handful of roughly chopped nuts and seeds if you don't have a batch on hand.

YIELD: 2 servings | **PREP TIME:** 5 minutes | **COOK TIME:** 0 minutes

1 cup whole-milk ricotta cheese

½ teaspoon citrus zest

1 tablespoon extra-virgin olive oil

3 to 4 drops liquid stevia

¼ cup citrus segments, from oranges, grapefruit, or blood orange

¼ cup Nut and Seed Granola with Olive Oil (page 13)

1. In a medium bowl, combine the ricotta, citrus zest, olive oil, and stevia. Divide between two serving bowls.
2. Top each bowl with a few citrus segments and 2 tablespoons of the granola.

NUTRITION PER SERVING

CALORIES: 394 TOTAL FAT: 34g PROTEIN: 16g CARBOHYDRATES: 8g FIBER: 2g NET CARBS: 6g

Macadamia Coconut Porridge DF GF Vg

If hot cereal is your jam, this version mimics the taste and texture of oatmeal. It's made with a blend of macadamia nuts, walnuts, and almonds. If you don't have one of them, feel free to double up on another. Ideally, soak the nuts overnight to soften, then rinse and drain before adding them to the recipe.

YIELD: 4 servings | **PREP TIME:** 5 minutes | **COOK TIME:** 3 minutes

- ½ cup macadamia nuts
- ½ cup walnuts
- ½ cup almonds
- 1 cup coconut milk
- 1 cup unsweetened almond milk
- 4 to 5 drops liquid stevia
- 1 teaspoon vanilla extract
- ½ teaspoon ground cinnamon
- ¼ teaspoon sea salt
- ¼ cup unsweetened shredded coconut, toasted

1. Place the macadamia nuts, walnuts, almonds, coconut milk, almond milk, stevia, vanilla, cinnamon, and salt in a blender and puree until mostly smooth. A little bit of texture is good.
2. Pour the mixture into a small saucepan and heat over medium-low heat until it begins to simmer.
3. Divide the mixture between serving bowls and top with the shredded coconut.

COOKING TIP: To toast the coconut, place it in a dry skillet over medium heat. Gently shake the pan as it cooks, until the coconut is evenly golden. Be careful not to burn.

NUTRITION PER SERVING

CALORIES: 467 **TOTAL FAT:** 46g **PROTEIN:** 9g **CARBOHYDRATES:** 12g **FIBER:** 6g **NET CARBS:** 6g

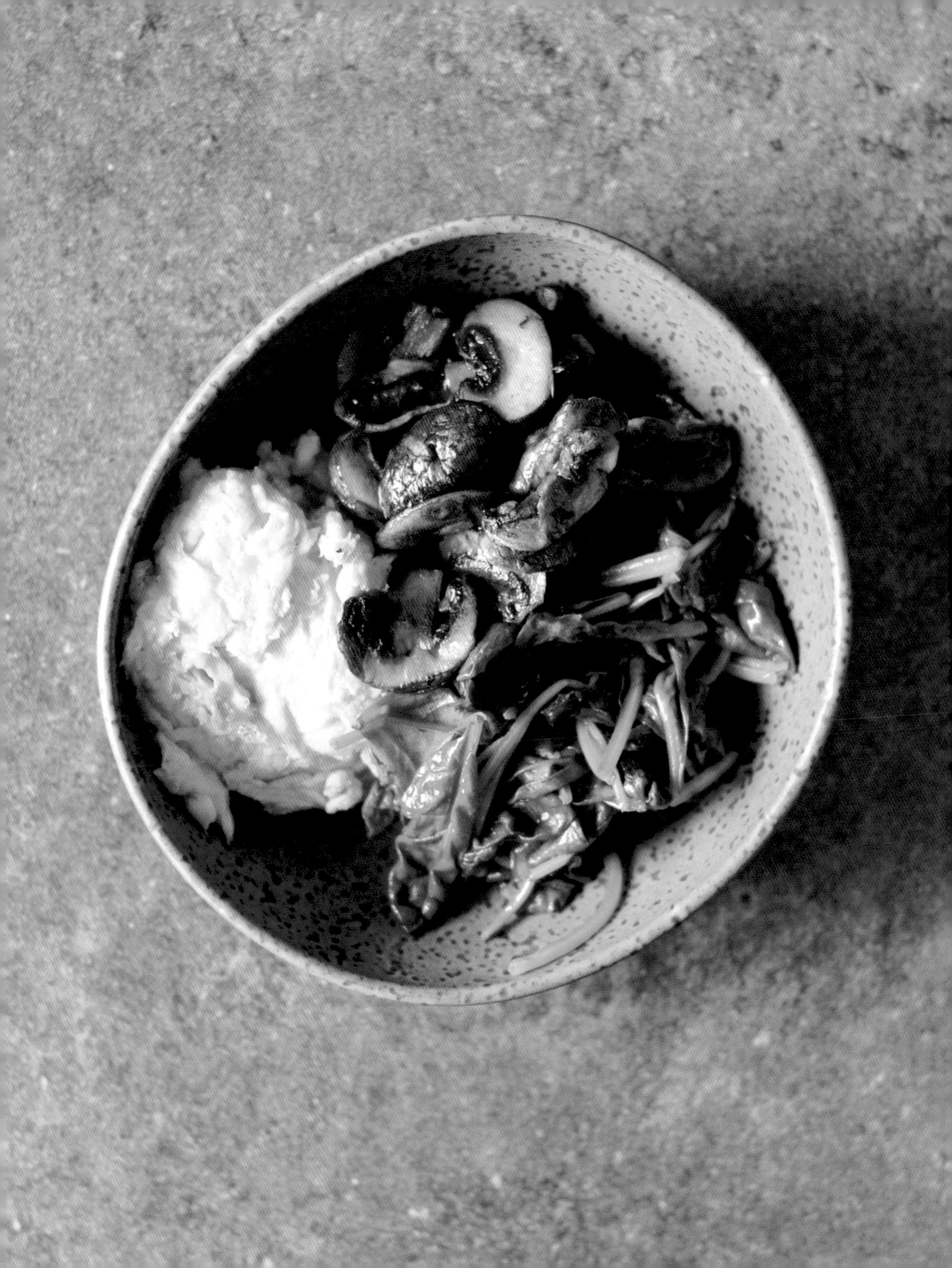

Rosemary Sautéed Mushrooms with Wilted Spinach and Scrambled Eggs GF NF V

This vegetarian deconstructed scramble gets complexity from the umami in the mushrooms and Parmesan, making it just as flavorful as any dish with meat. While you can certainly mix it all together, I prefer to keep the individual ingredients separated because I think it's prettier that way and the texture of the scrambled eggs is better without the addition of spinach, which seeps moisture.

YIELD: 1 serving | **PREP TIME:** 5 minutes | **COOK TIME:** 11 minutes

- 1 tablespoon olive oil, divided
- 1 tablespoon butter
- 1 cup sliced mushrooms
- 1 teaspoon minced fresh rosemary
- 2 cups packed spinach
- 1 small clove garlic, minced
- 2 eggs, whisked
- sea salt
- freshly ground pepper
- ¼ cup grated Parmesan

1. Heat a medium skillet over medium-high heat. Add ½ tablespoon olive oil and butter. When it's melted, add the mushrooms and rosemary, and sauté until well browned and soft, about 5 minutes. Transfer the mushrooms to the serving dish.
2. Add the spinach and garlic to the pan and cook until the spinach begins to wilt but is not losing water, about 1 minute. Transfer to the serving dish.
3. Reduce the heat to medium-low. Add the remaining ½ tablespoon olive oil to the pan and cook the eggs until just set, about 5 minutes. Season with salt and pepper. Stir in the Parmesan. Transfer to the serving dish and serve immediately.

NUTRITION PER SERVING

CALORIES: 485 TOTAL FAT: 41g PROTEIN: 25g CARBOHYDRATES: 6g FIBER: 2g NET CARBS: 4g

BLT Scramble Bowl DF GF NF

If you've been keto for any length of time—heck, even five minutes—you already have bacon and eggs down pat. Here's a way to liven up a classic combo inspired by the BLT. I add avocado to the bacon, lettuce, and tomato and swap the bread for eggs.

YIELD: 1 serving | **PREP TIME:** 5 minutes | **COOK TIME:** 17 minutes

2 slices applewood-smoked bacon, halved

1 green onion, white and green parts, thinly sliced

2 eggs, whisked

¼ cup grape tomatoes, halved

½ avocado, sliced

handful of chopped lettuce

1. Place the bacon slices in a small skillet. Cook over medium-low heat until crisp-tender, about 10 minutes. Set on a cooling rack to crisp up.
2. Add the green onion to the pan and cook for about 2 minutes, until they begin to soften.
3. Add the eggs to the pan and stir slowly until just set, about 5 minutes.
4. Place the scramble into a bowl. Top with the bacon, tomatoes, avocado, and lettuce.

INGREDIENT TIP: Avocados have a surprising amount of carbohydrates, given that they're the darlings of the keto community. But don't worry—more than 90 percent of those carbs are soluble and insoluble fiber, which is easy to skimp on in a low-carb diet.

NUTRITION PER SERVING

CALORIES: 44 TOTAL FAT: 35g PROTEIN: 21g CARBOHYDRATES: 13g FIBER: 7g NET CARBS: 6g

Roasted Vegetables and Sausage with Eggs and Sriracha DF GF NF

I'm a sucker for sheet pan recipes and even wrote a couple of books devoted to the concept. Because you're going to heat up the oven anyway, you may as well roast a few portions. They're great over salad or topped with eggs, as in this recipe. They also freeze well or can be folded into a scramble.

YIELD: 4 servings | **PREP TIME:** 10 minutes | **COOK TIME:** 45 minutes

- 1 small bunch broccoli, cut into florets
- 1 medium zucchini, cut into 1-inch pieces
- ½ medium onion, sliced into 8 wedges
- 1 large red bell pepper, cored and sliced into spears
- 1 pound Italian pork sausage (mild or hot), cut into 1-inch pieces
- 1½ tablespoons canola oil, divided
- sea salt
- freshly ground pepper
- 4 eggs
- sriracha, for serving

1. Preheat the oven to 375°F. Line a rimmed baking sheet with parchment paper.
2. Spread the broccoli, zucchini, onion, pepper, and sausage onto the prepared pan. Drizzle with ½ tablespoon canola oil and season generously with salt and pepper.
3. Roast for 30 minutes. Stir the ingredients and return to the oven for another 10 minutes until gently browned.
4. Meanwhile, to prepare the eggs, heat 1 tablespoon canola oil in a large skillet over medium-high heat. Fry the eggs until the whites are completely set, about 5 minutes. Season with salt and pepper.
5. Divide the vegetables and sausage between serving dishes. Top each with two fried eggs and drizzle with sriracha.

FREEZER FRIENDLY: Allow the cooked tray to cool completely then transfer to the freezer. Freeze until solid and then divide into storage containers, either zip-top plastic bags or meal-prep containers.

NUTRITION PER SERVING

CALORIES: 426 TOTAL FAT: 33g PROTEIN: 25g CARBOHYDRATES: 7g FIBER: 2g NET CARBS: 5g

Smoked Salmon and Spinach Scramble DF GF NF

When I prepared this recipe, I used smoked salmon from Lummi Island provided by Patagonia Provisions. I grew up vacationing and playing in Lummi's icy waters. My family always caught Dungeness crab, which also goes well in this bowl. This healthy, colorful breakfast comes together quickly, so be sure to have all of the ingredients prepped ahead of time.

YIELD: 1 serving | **PREP TIME:** 5 minutes | **COOK TIME:** 5 minutes

1 tablespoon canola oil

1 green onion, white and green parts, thinly sliced

2 eggs

1 packed cup fresh spinach

2 ounces smoked salmon

1 small avocado, sliced

1. Heat a small skillet over medium-high heat. Add the canola oil and tilt to coat the bottom of the pan. Add the white parts of the chopped green onions and cook until they begin to brown, stirring frequently, about 2 minutes.
2. Add the eggs and cook for about 1 minute, or until nearly set.
3. Fold the spinach into the eggs and cook for about 30 seconds, just until the spinach begins to wilt. Remove the pan from the heat.
4. Fold the smoked salmon in gently, being careful not to break it up too much.
5. To serve, top the scramble with the remaining sliced green onions and the avocado.

NUTRITION PER SERVING

CALORIES: 423 **TOTAL FAT:** 33g **PROTEIN:** 25g **CARBOHYDRATES:** 7g **FIBER:** 5g **NET CARBS:** 2g

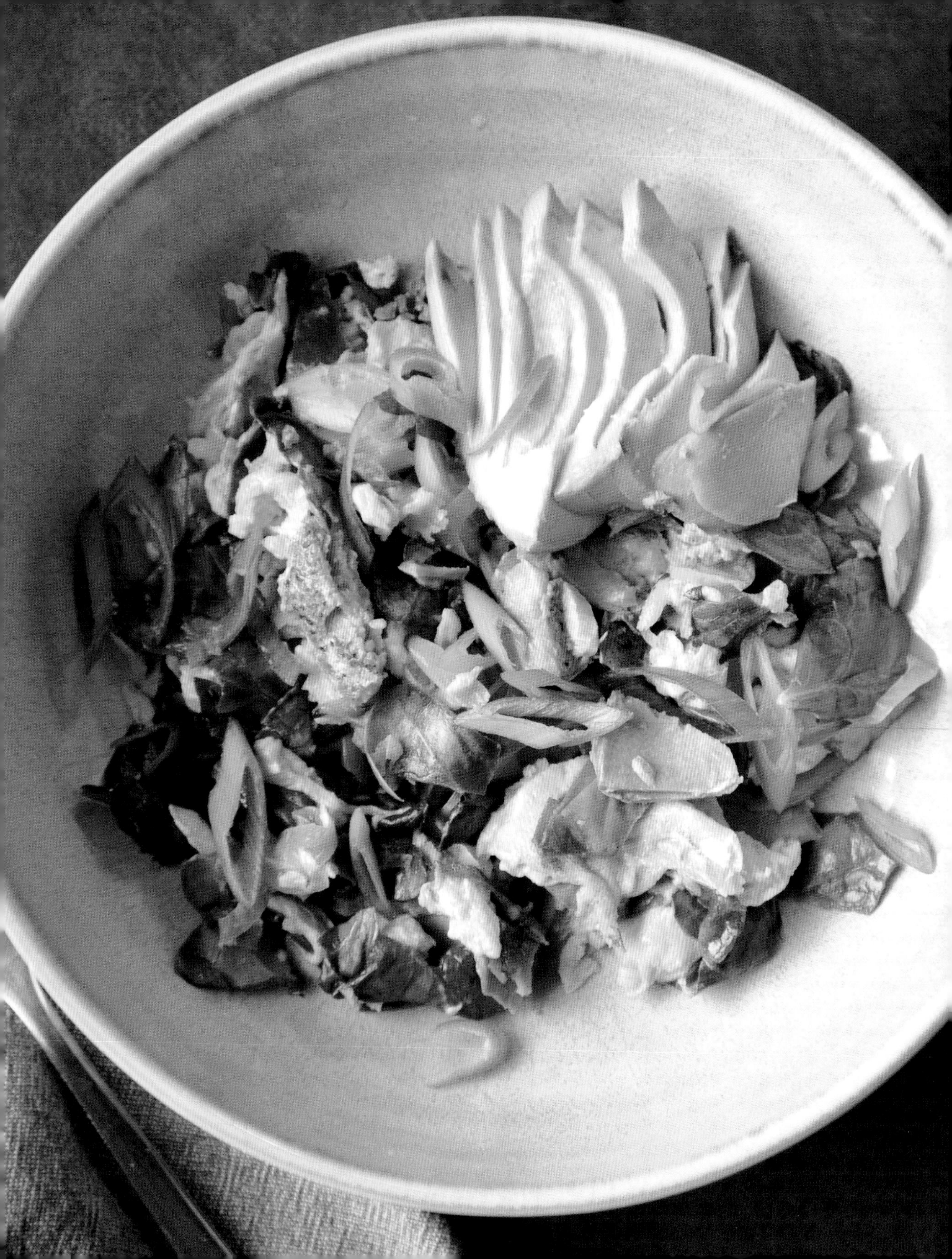

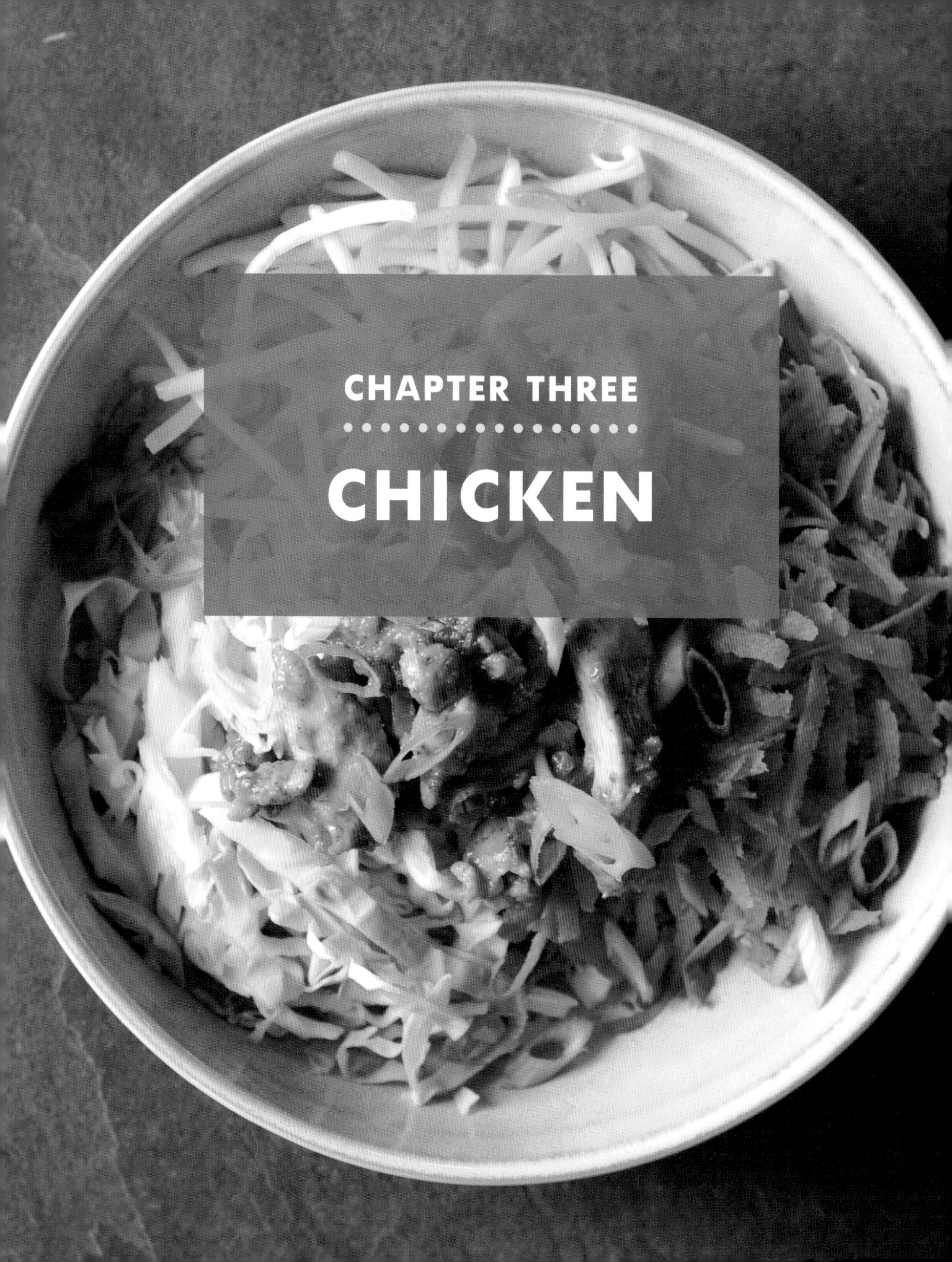

CHAPTER THREE

CHICKEN

Chicken can easily become a routine staple in your low-carb kitchen. I've livened it up with flavor and inspiration from around the globe. Start with the Adobo Chicken with Seared Bok Choy—it'll knock your socks off. Then give the Smoky Chicken and Broccoli Bowls a try—they're reminiscent of the ubiquitous mid-century potluck broccoli salads but with a little more bulk to make them a meal.

- Green Goddess Chicken with Jicama Noodles
- Pesto Zucchini Noodles with Chicken
- Chicken Burrito Bowls
- Adobo Chicken with Seared Bok Choy
- Thai Peanut Chicken with Carrot and Cabbage Slaw
- Sesame Ginger Chicken Salad
- Roasted Chicken over Cauliflower Puree with Wilted Greens
- Smoky Chicken and Broccoli Bowls

Green Goddess Chicken with Jicama Noodles DF GF NF

Of all the fun vegetables to spiralize, jicama is in my top three. Because of its wide shape, it easily makes long strands that are fun to twirl around a fork. I also love its crunchy texture, a nice contrast to the tangy green goddess chicken.

YIELD: 4 servings | **PREP TIME:** 10 minutes | **COOK TIME:** 0 minutes

GREEN GODDESS DRESSING

¼ cup minced fresh parsley

½ cup roughly chopped fresh basil

¼ cup minced fresh chives

2 cups baby spinach

½ tablespoon apple cider vinegar

1 teaspoon lemon juice

1 teaspoon Dijon mustard

½ teaspoon sea salt

¾ cup mayonnaise

3 cups shredded or diced cooked chicken

1 small jicama (about 1 pound), peeled and spiralized

2 green onions, white and green parts, thinly sliced

1 cup romaine or iceberg lettuce, shredded

1. To make the green goddess dressing, combine the parsley, basil, chives, baby spinach, apple cider vinegar, lemon juice, mustard, sea salt, and mayonnaise in a blender. Puree until smooth.
2. In a small bowl, combine the chicken with the green goddess dressing. Set aside.
3. To serve, divide the spiralized jicama between serving dishes. Top with the chicken, green onions, and lettuce.

NUTRITION PER SERVING

CALORIES: 478 TOTAL FAT: 35g PROTEIN: 30g CARBOHYDRATES: 11g FIBER: 6g NET CARBS: 5g

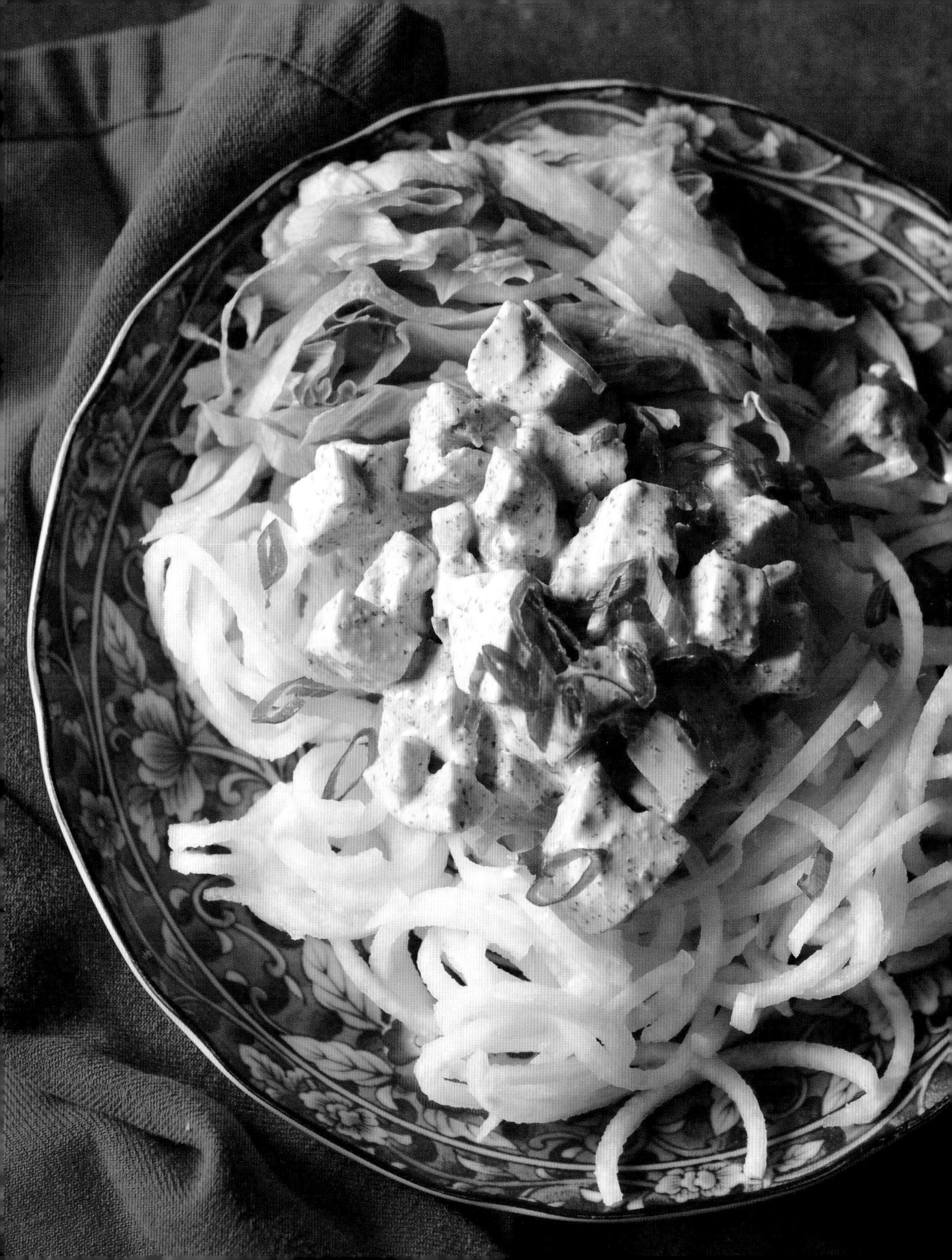

Pesto Zucchini Noodles with Chicken GF

If you want simplicity, this instant classic has it. It takes just a handful of familiar ingredients and creates a colorful keto meal in minutes.

YIELD: 2 servings | **PREP TIME:** 10 minutes | **COOK TIME:** 5 minutes

4 medium zucchini, spiralized
sea salt
1 tablespoon extra-virgin olive oil
1 cup prepared pesto
3 cups shredded or diced cooked chicken
2 tablespoons toasted pine nuts
2 tablespoons grated Parmesan
½ cup halved grape tomatoes
shredded basil, for garnish

1. Prepare the zucchini according to the instructions for Vegetable Noodles on page 103.
2. Heat a large skillet over medium-high heat. When it's hot, add the olive oil.
3. Sauté the zucchini for 3 minutes, or until just heated through.
4. Reduce the heat to low and stir in the pesto and chicken. Cook until just heated through, about 1 minute.
5. Transfer the pasta to a serving dish. Top with the pine nuts, Parmesan, grape tomatoes, and basil.

NUTRITION PER SERVING

CALORIES: 594 TOTAL FAT: 46g PROTEIN: 35g CARBOHYDRATES: 13g FIBER: 3g NET CARBS: 10g

Chicken Burrito Bowls DF GF NF

Living in California means living with some pretty epic Mexican food—slow-cooked barbacoa, brilliant pico de gallo, and fiery homemade salsas. I've tried to capture some of my favorite flavors in this burrito bowl. Noticeably absent from the recipe are beans, rice, and a tortilla and a ton of carbs, but you won't miss them! The dish takes a bit of time to prepare, but I've designed the recipe to yield four portions, so you can meal prep.

YIELD: 4 servings | **PREP TIME:** 10 minutes | **COOK TIME:** 10 to 14 minutes

- 2 large cloves garlic, minced
- 1 teaspoon sea salt
- 2 teaspoons ground coriander
- 2 tablespoons ground cumin
- 2 tablespoons smoked paprika
- 2 tablespoons extra-virgin olive oil, divided
- 4 bone-in, skin-on chicken thighs
- ½ cup crushed tomatoes
- 4 cups shredded romaine lettuce
- ¼ cup roughly chopped cilantro
- 1 cup pico de gallo salsa
- 1 cup Guacamole (page 104) or store-bought guacamole

1. Combine the garlic, salt, coriander, cumin, paprika, and 1 tablespoon of the olive oil in a small bowl. Coat the chicken thighs with this mixture. If you have time, place the chicken thighs in a zip-top plastic bag and let them marinate overnight.
2. Heat a large skillet over medium-high heat. Add the remaining tablespoon of olive oil. Sear the chicken, skin-side down until well browned, 5 to 7 minutes.
3. Flip the chicken, add the crushed tomatoes, reduce the heat to medium, and cover the pan with a lid. Cook for 5 to 7 minutes, or until the chicken is cooked through. When it is cool enough to handle, shred the chicken right into the pan. Discard the bones.
4. Divide the lettuce between serving bowls. Top with the cooked chicken, cilantro, pico de gallo, and guacamole.

INGREDIENT TIP: Not to be confused with cilantro, coriander is the seed of the plant. You can find it in the spices section. Like peppercorns, it must be ground before using (except when it is removed from the finished dish before serving).

NUTRITION PER SERVING

CALORIES: 360 TOTAL FAT: 22g PROTEIN: 30g CARBOHYDRATES: 9g FIBER: 6g NET CARBS: 3g

Adobo Chicken with Seared Bok Choy DF NF

When I was in college, I worked for an Asian newspaper in Portland. The owners are Filipino and often cooked adobo chicken and pork for lunches—talk about benefits! The fragrant aromas filled the office, making it almost impossible to get anything done. This version of adobo chicken is served over cauliflower rice with seared bok choy for a healthier and much lower-carb meal.

YIELD: 4 servings | **PREP TIME:** 10 minutes | **COOK TIME:** 30 minutes

- 1½ pounds boneless, skinless chicken thighs, cut into 2-inch pieces
- 1 cup distilled white vinegar
- ½ cup low-sodium soy sauce
- 2 cloves garlic, crushed
- 2 bay leaves
- 1 teaspoon peppercorns
- 2 tablespoons canola oil
- 4 heads baby bok choy
- 1 recipe Cauli Rice (page 100)
- 2 green onions, white and green parts, thinly sliced
- 1 tablespoon sesame seeds

1. Place the chicken, vinegar, soy sauce, garlic, bay leaves, and peppercorns into a large pot and bring to a simmer over medium heat. Cover and cook for 15 minutes. Remove the chicken to a separate dish.
2. Continue simmering the sauce uncovered for another 15 minutes until it's reduced by half. It should be about ¾ cup.
3. Meanwhile, heat a large skillet over medium-high heat. Add the canola oil to the hot pan. Add the bok choy to the pan cut-side down and sear until deeply browned, 3 to 4 minutes. Flip over and brown on the other side for 2 minutes.
4. To serve, divide the cauliflower rice between serving bowls. Top with the chicken, bok choy, green onions, and sesame seeds.

INGREDIENT TIP: It's especially important to use low-sodium soy sauce here. Otherwise the sauce ends up way too salty.

NUTRITION PER SERVING

CALORIES: 382 TOTAL FAT: 19g PROTEIN: 41g CARBOHYDRATES: 13g FIBER: 7g NET CARBS: 6g

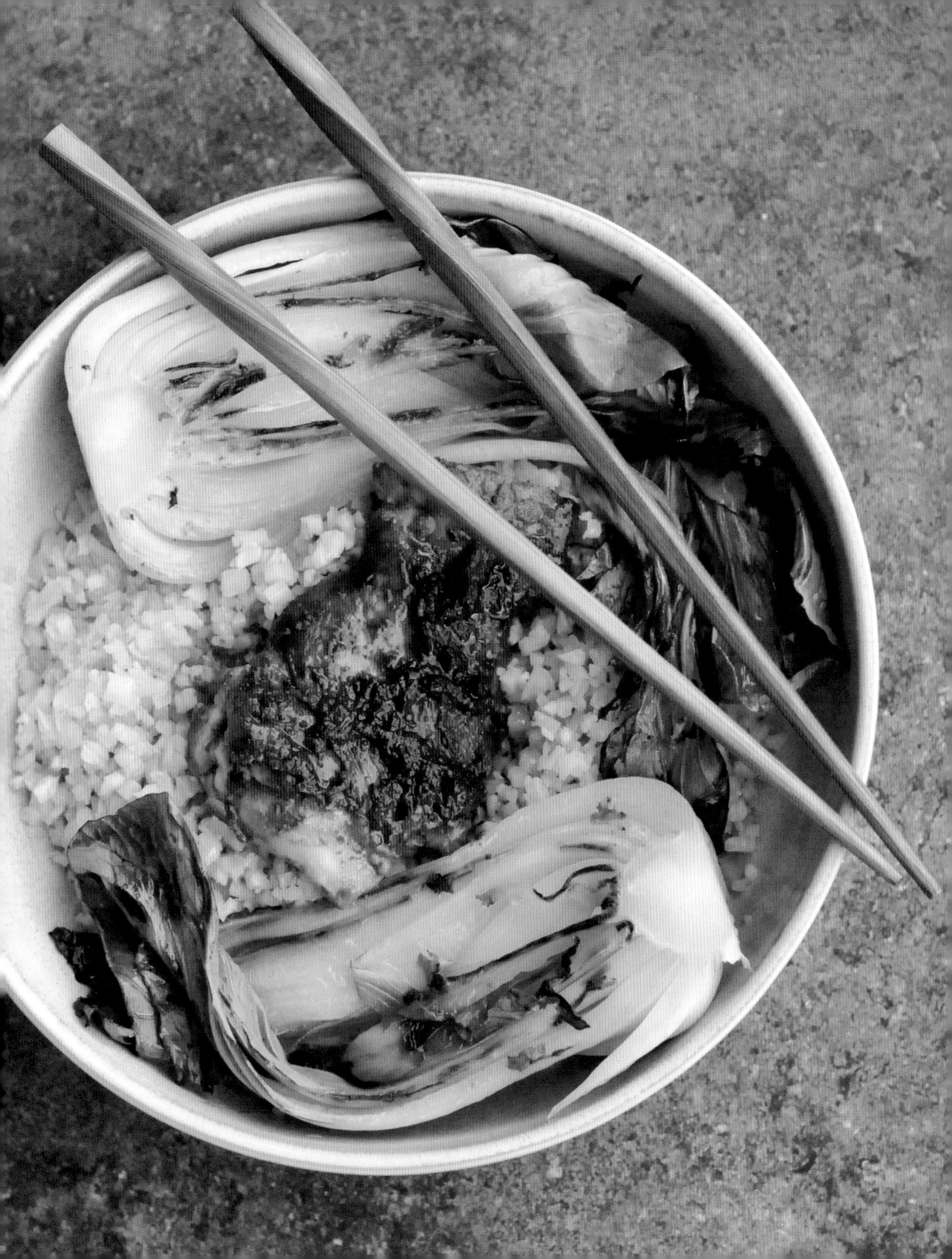

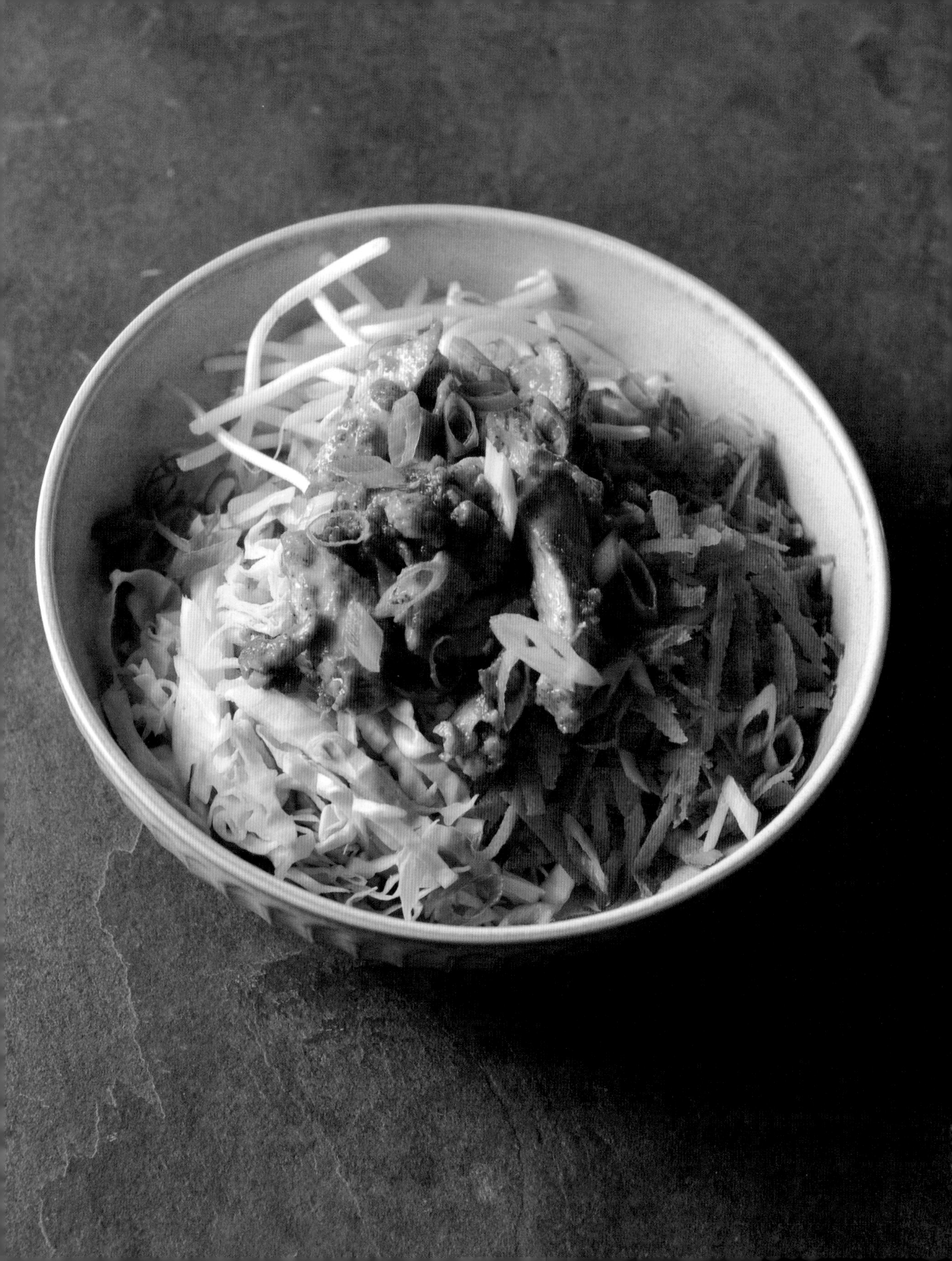

Thai Peanut Chicken with Carrot and Cabbage Slaw DF GF

Peanut sauce is my undoing. Like most Thai food, it presents the perfect balance of salty, sweet, sour, spicy, and savory. If you don't have fish sauce, or aren't keen on its pungent aroma, you can use soy sauce.

YIELD: 4 servings | **PREP TIME:** 10 minutes | **COOK TIME:** 8 to 10 minutes

- 2 tablespoons canola oil
- 1½ pounds boneless, skinless chicken thighs
- 1 tablespoon minced ginger
- 1 teaspoon minced garlic
- ¼ teaspoon red chili flakes
- 1 tablespoon fish sauce
- ½ cup natural peanut butter
- 1 tablespoon lime juice
- ¼ cup water
- 1 to 2 drops liquid stevia
- 2 cups shredded cabbage
- 1 cup bean sprouts
- 2 green onions, white and green parts, thinly sliced
- 1 carrot, peeled, cut into matchsticks or spiralized
- sea salt

1. Heat a large skillet over medium-high heat. Add the canola oil and tilt to coat the pan.
2. Pat the chicken dry with paper towels and then season generously with salt. Sear for 4 to 5 minutes on each side, or until cooked through. Transfer to a separate dish.
3. Add the ginger, garlic, and red chili flakes to the pan and cook for 30 seconds. Add the fish sauce and simmer for about 30 seconds.
4. Stir in the peanut butter, lime juice, and water. Whisk to form a sauce, adding additional water as needed until it reaches the desired consistency, about 2 minutes. Add 1 to 2 drops liquid stevia, to taste.
5. Divide the cabbage, bean sprouts, green onions, and carrot between serving bowls. Top with the chicken and drizzle with peanut sauce.

COOKING TIP: For meal prepping, place the chicken and salad next to each other in a meal-prep container and keep the sauce in a separate small container.

NUTRITION PER SERVING

CALORIES: 478 TOTAL FAT: 30g PROTEIN: 43g CARBOHYDRATES: 12g FIBER: 4g NET CARBS: 8g

Sesame Ginger Chicken Salad DF NF

Toasted sesame oil, soy sauce, lime juice, and pungent ginger and garlic permeate the dressing in this simple Asian chicken salad.

YIELD: 4 servings | **PREP TIME:** 10 minutes | **COOK TIME:** 0 minutes

2 tablespoons toasted sesame oil

2 tablespoons canola oil

2 tablespoons soy sauce

1 tablespoon lime juice

1 teaspoon minced fresh ginger

1 teaspoon minced fresh garlic

pinch of red chili flakes

4 cups shredded cabbage

¼ cup roughly chopped cilantro

¼ cup roughly chopped mint

1 pound shredded, cooked chicken breasts

1 green onion, white and green parts, thinly sliced

4 tablespoons sesame seeds

1. Whisk together the sesame oil, canola oil, soy sauce, lime juice, ginger, garlic, and red chili flakes in a medium salad bowl.
2. Add the cabbage, cilantro, mint, and green onion to the bowl and toss gently to mix. Sprinkle with the sesame seeds before serving.

COOKING TIP: Use store-bought chicken for this recipe and shred using two forks. To prepare it from raw chicken, coat bone-in chicken breasts with a teaspoon of oil, season with salt and pepper, and roast in a 400°F oven for 30 minutes, or until the juices run clear. When cool enough to handle, shred using two forks.

NUTRITION PER SERVING

CALORIES: 337 FAT: 22g PROTEIN: 29g TOTAL CARBS: 8g FIBER: 4g NET CARBS: 4g

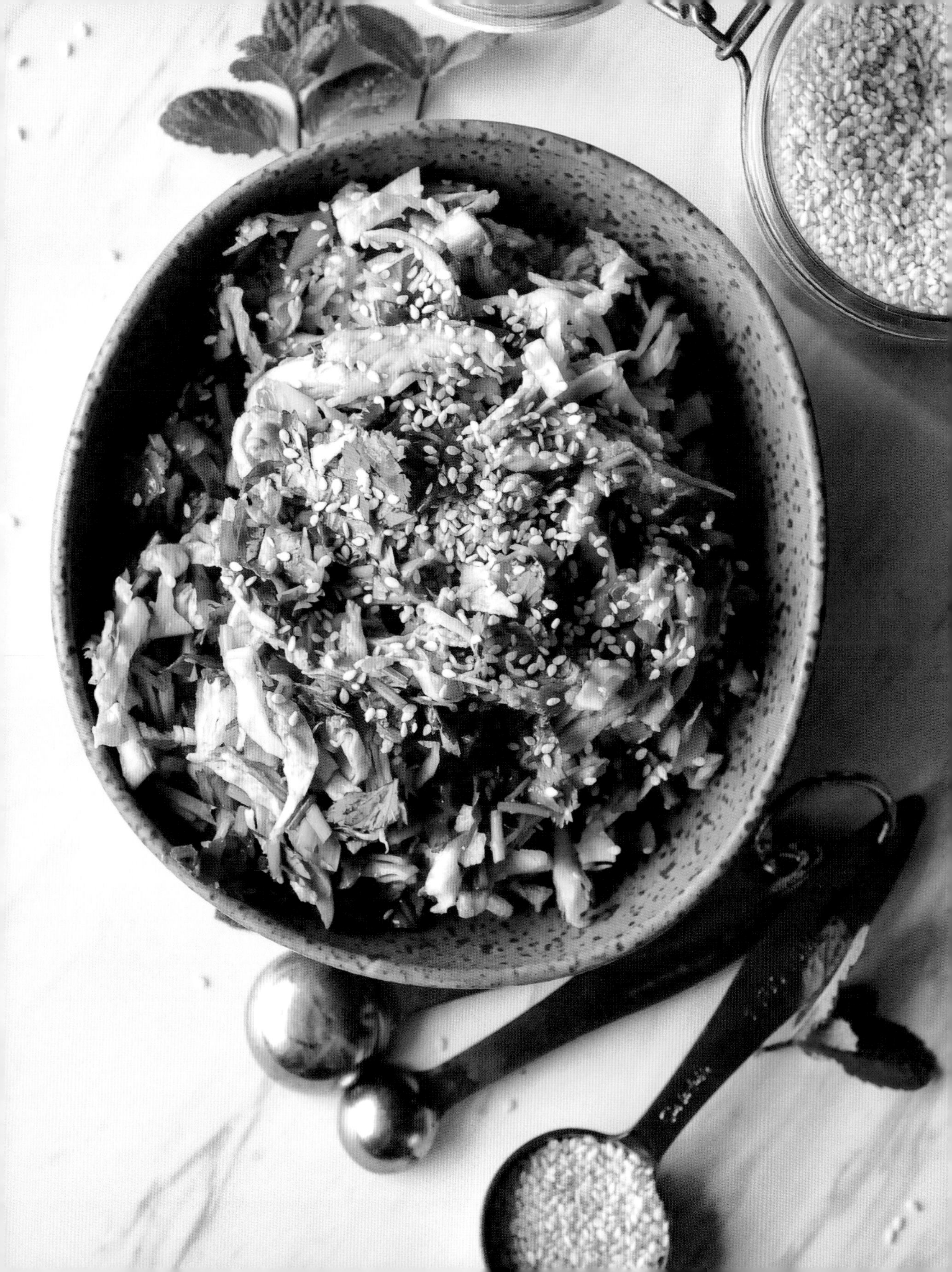

Roasted Chicken over Cauliflower Puree with Wilted Greens GF NF

When I think of bowl meals, my mind goes one of two places—either bright, fresh, and crunchy salad bowls with lots of raw veggies and a tangy dressing or thick, rich, creamy comfort food dishes with roasted meat and cooked vegetables. This dish is decidedly in the latter camp. It calls for bone-in chicken legs, but if you prefer boneless, that's fine too; simply use two chicken thighs.

YIELD: 4 servings | **PREP TIME:** 5 minutes | **COOK TIME:** 27 minutes

- 1 tablespoon canola oil
- 4 bone-in, skin-on chicken leg quarters (the leg and thigh)
- sea salt
- freshly ground pepper
- 1 sprig thyme
- 8 packed cups spinach
- 1 teaspoon minced garlic
- 2 teaspoons balsamic vinegar
- 1 recipe Mashed Cauliflower (page 98)

1. Preheat the oven to 400°F. Heat a large, ovenproof skillet, such as cast iron, over medium-high heat. When it's hot, add the oil.
2. Pat the chicken legs dry with paper towels and season generously with salt and pepper. Place them skin-side down into the pan and sear for 5 minutes. Flip the chicken, add the thyme, then transfer the pan to the oven. Roast for 20 minutes, or until cooked through.
3. Carefully return the pan to the stovetop. Transfer the cooked chicken to a separate dish to rest.
4. Add the spinach and garlic to the pan and cook until the spinach begins to wilt, about 1 minute. Add the balsamic vinegar and cook until all of the greens are soft, 30 to 60 seconds more.
5. Divide the mashed cauliflower between serving bowls. Top with the wilted spinach and a chicken leg.

NUTRITION PER SERVING

CALORIES: 547 TOTAL FAT: 37g PROTEIN: 47g CARBOHYDRATES: 10g FIBER: 5g NET CARBS: 5g

Smoky Chicken and Broccoli Bowls DF GF

Broccoli salad is almost a meal and it's tasty enough that most of the time I wish it were. This version gets a protein boost from shredded chicken.

YIELD: 4 servings | **PREP TIME:** 10 minutes | **COOK TIME:** 10 minutes

- 2 slices applewood-smoked bacon, cut into pieces
- ½ cup mayonnaise
- juice of 1 lemon
- sea salt
- freshly ground pepper
- 4 cups raw broccoli florets
- ½ small red onion, thinly sliced
- 1 cup shredded red cabbage
- 2 cups shredded cooked chicken breasts
- ¼ cup roughly chopped toasted almonds

1. Cook the bacon in a medium skillet over medium-low heat until the bacon is crisp and has rendered most of its fat, about 10 minutes. Set the bacon aside.
2. Pour the bacon fat into a large salad bowl. Add the mayonnaise and lemon juice and whisk to combine. Season with salt and pepper.
3. Add the broccoli, onion, red cabbage, and chicken to the bowl and coat thoroughly. Divide between serving bowls.
4. Sprinkle the bacon pieces and toasted almonds over the salad just before serving.

NUTRITION PER SERVING

CALORIES: 422 FAT: 29g PROTEIN: 32g TOTAL CARBS: 10g FIBER: 5g NET CARBS: 5g

CHAPTER FOUR

FISH & SEAFOOD

Having grown up in the Pacific Northwest, seafood is deeply embedded in my culinary heritage. I watched salmon leap up fish ladders in the Columbia Gorge, caught Dungeness crab in the icy waters off the San Juan Islands, and learned to love clams and mussels while working in restaurants in Portland. If you're not normally a "fish person" I hope you'll give these recipes a shot. Start with the coconut salmon. It's savory and sweet and might just make you rethink seafood.

- Coconut Salmon with Roasted Cauliflower and Asparagus
- Seared Salmon and Broccoli Mash
- Niçoise Salad Bowls
- Poke Bowls with Avocado and Sesame Seeds
- Paella with Cauli Rice
- Spicy Mussels with Roasted Fennel and Tomatoes
- Grilled Swordfish with Caper Gremolata

Coconut Salmon with Roasted Cauliflower and Asparagus DF GF NF

Many bowl meals require a lot of separate recipes. Not this one! This one-pan meal has it all—creamy baked salmon, crunchy roasted cauliflower, and tender asparagus. Finish things off with a tangy ginger coconut sauce.

YIELD: 4 servings | **PREP TIME:** 10 minutes | **COOK TIME:** 25 to 27 minutes

1 small head cauliflower, broken into florets
1 teaspoon curry powder
2 tablespoons melted coconut oil, divided
1 bunch asparagus
sea salt
½ cup coconut cream
1 tablespoon fish sauce
1 teaspoon minced ginger
zest and juice of 1 lime
1 to 2 drops liquid stevia
1 pound salmon
handful of fresh cilantro

1. Preheat the oven to 400°F. Line a sheet pan with parchment paper.
2. Spread the cauliflower out on the baking sheet, sprinkle with the curry powder, season with salt, and add 1 tablespoon of the coconut oil, and toss gently to mix. Roast for 10 minutes.
3. Meanwhile, coat the asparagus with the remaining tablespoon of coconut oil. Season with salt. Push the cauliflower to one side of the baking sheet. Spread the asparagus onto the sheet pan and roast for another 10 minutes.
4. While the asparagus cooks, pour the coconut cream, fish sauce, ginger, lime zest and juice, and liquid stevia into a small jar. Cover with a lid and shake vigorously to combine.
5. Place the salmon onto the sheet pan, pushing the other vegetables to the sides. Brush with half of the coconut mixture. Bake for 5 to 7 minutes, or until the salmon flakes easily with a fork.
6. Divide the cauliflower and asparagus between four serving bowls. Top with the salmon. Drizzle with the remaining coconut sauce and garnish with cilantro.

NUTRITION PER SERVING

CALORIES: 389 TOTAL FAT: 23g PROTEIN: 37g CARBOHYDRATES: 8g FIBER: 4g NET CARBS: 4g

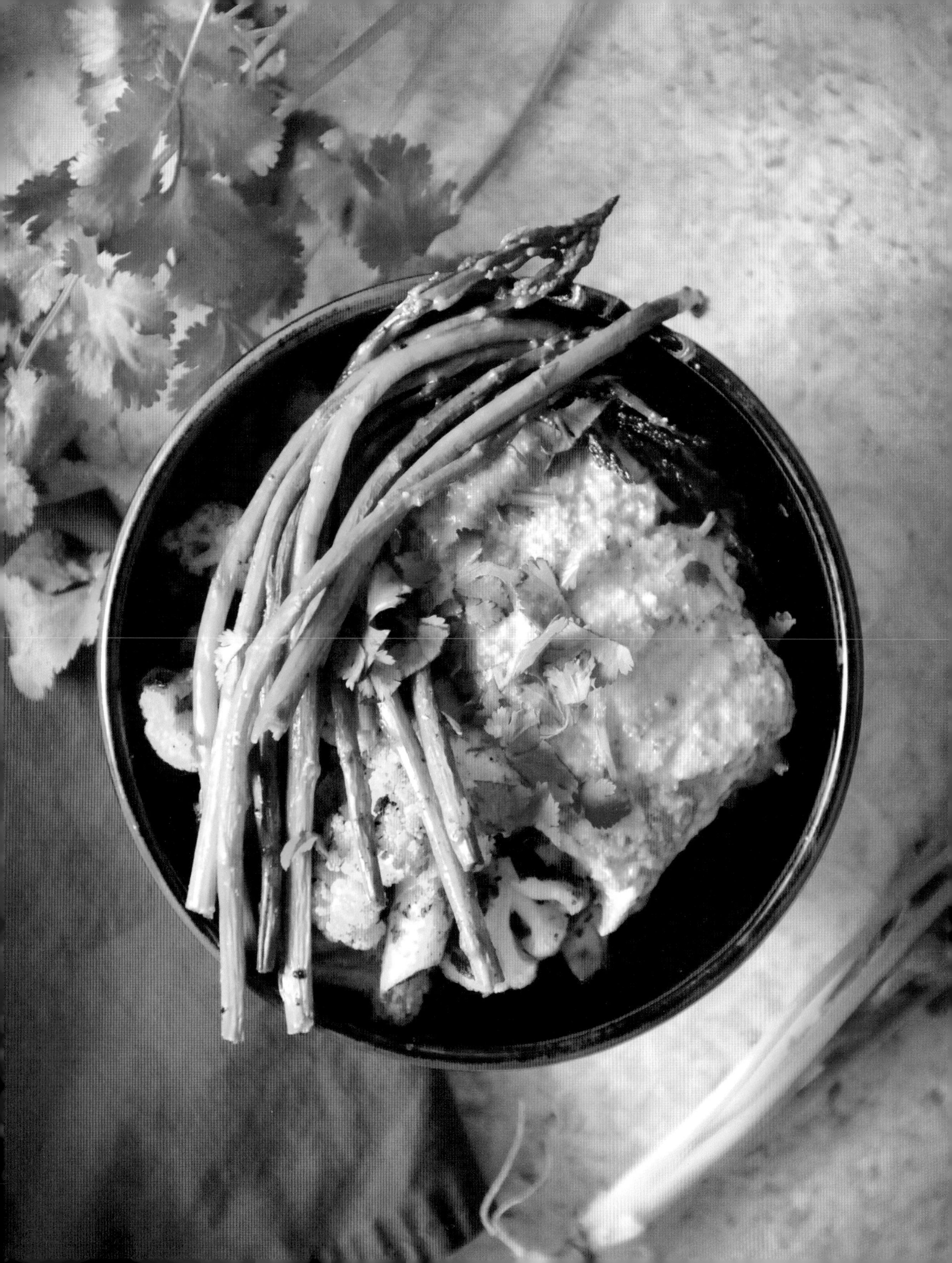

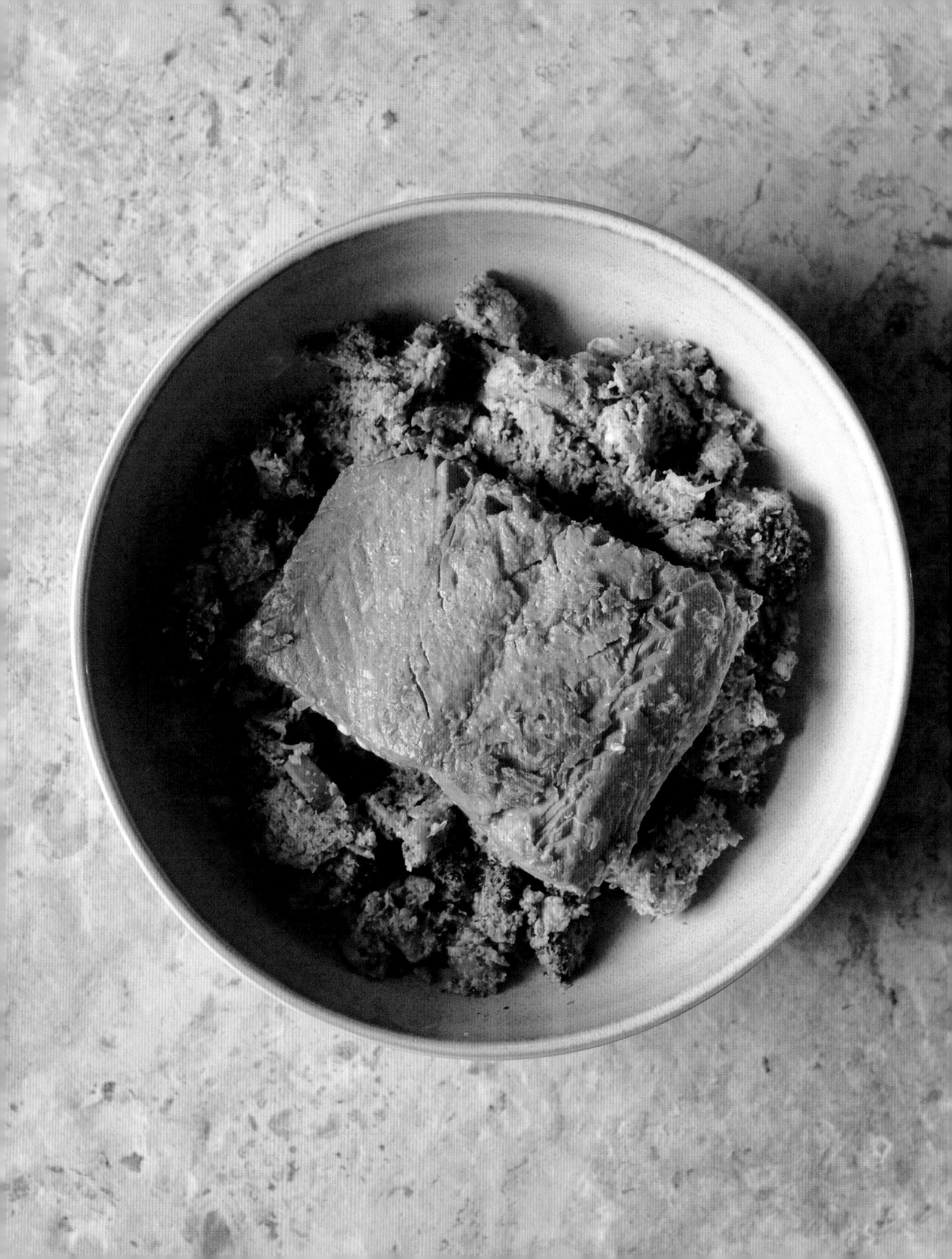

Seared Salmon and Broccoli Mash GF NF

If you can make mashed cauliflower, why not broccoli? It's green, sure, so it doesn't do a very good job of pretending to be mashed potatoes. But that's okay—it's so delicious, it doesn't matter. I've tried to keep this bowl ultra-simple because sometimes you just need a healthy keto meal without having to empty your pantry.

YIELD: 4 servings | **PREP TIME:** 5 minutes | **COOK TIME:** 20 minutes

3 tablespoons extra-virgin olive oil, divided
1 head broccoli, cut into florets
2 teaspoons minced garlic
pinch of red chili flakes
½ cup chicken broth
½ cup plain, whole-milk yogurt
1 pound salmon
sea salt

1. Heat 2 tablespoons of the oil in a large skillet over medium-high heat until hot. Add the broccoli and allow to cook undisturbed for 3 minutes, or until well browned.
2. Add the garlic and red chili flakes and cook for 30 seconds, until just fragrant. Add the chicken broth. Cover and simmer for 15 minutes, or until the broccoli is tender.
3. Add the yogurt and use an immersion blender to break up the broccoli until it's still somewhat chunky.
4. While the broccoli cooks, heat the remaining tablespoon of oil in a large skillet over medium-high heat until hot. Season the salmon with salt. Sear on each side for 2 to 3 minutes, until it reaches your desired level of doneness. Remember, it will continue cooking once you remove it from the heat.
5. Divide the mashed broccoli between serving plates and top with the salmon.

NUTRITION PER SERVING

CALORIES: 320 TOTAL FAT: 17g PROTEIN: 35g CARBOHYDRATES: 9g FIBER: 5g NET CARBS: 4g

Niçoise Salad Bowls DF GF NF

Everyone claims an authentic variation of Niçoise salad, a French classic. I make no claims other than that it is a light, refreshing, and healthy keto salad. I'll admit, this recipe does involve a few steps, but once you have everything in place, it doesn't really take that long to execute. It makes an excellent meal prep dish, so you can put that work to use for a couple days. I kept the portion sizes small, but you could easily split this between two people.

YIELD: 4 servings | **PREP TIME:** 10 minutes | **COOK TIME:** 20 minutes

- 8 ounces green beans
- 8 eggs
- 8 ounces ahi tuna
- ¼ cup extra-virgin olive oil, plus more for fish
- sea salt
- freshly ground pepper
- 2 tablespoons white wine vinegar
- 1 teaspoon Dijon mustard
- 1 shallot, minced
- 8 cups mixed baby lettuces
- ½ cup Niçoise olives
- 1 cup halved grape or cherry tomatoes

1. Bring a large pot of salted water to a boil. Blanch the green beans, cooking for 3 to 5 minutes, or until bright green and crisp-tender. Transfer to a colander and rinse under cold water or chill in an ice-water bath.
2. Place the eggs into the boiling water, cover the pot, and remove the pot from the heat. Cook in the water for 12 minutes. Transfer to an ice-water bath and then peel and cut in half.
3. While the eggs cook, heat a large skillet over medium-high heat. Pat the tuna dry with paper towels then coat lightly in olive oil. Season with salt and pepper. Sear the tuna for about 90 seconds on each side. Transfer to a cutting board and then cut into ½-inch-thick slices.
4. In a large bowl, whisk the vinegar, mustard, shallot, and olive oil until emulsified. Season with salt and pepper.
5. Add the lettuce and green beans to the bowl and toss gently to coat.
6. Divide the dressed vegetables between serving bowls. Top each with eggs, a few slices of tuna, olives, and a few tomatoes.

NUTRITION PER SERVING

CALORIES: 367 TOTAL FAT: 27g PROTEIN: 20g CARBOHYDRATES: 14g FIBER: 3g NET CARBS: 11g

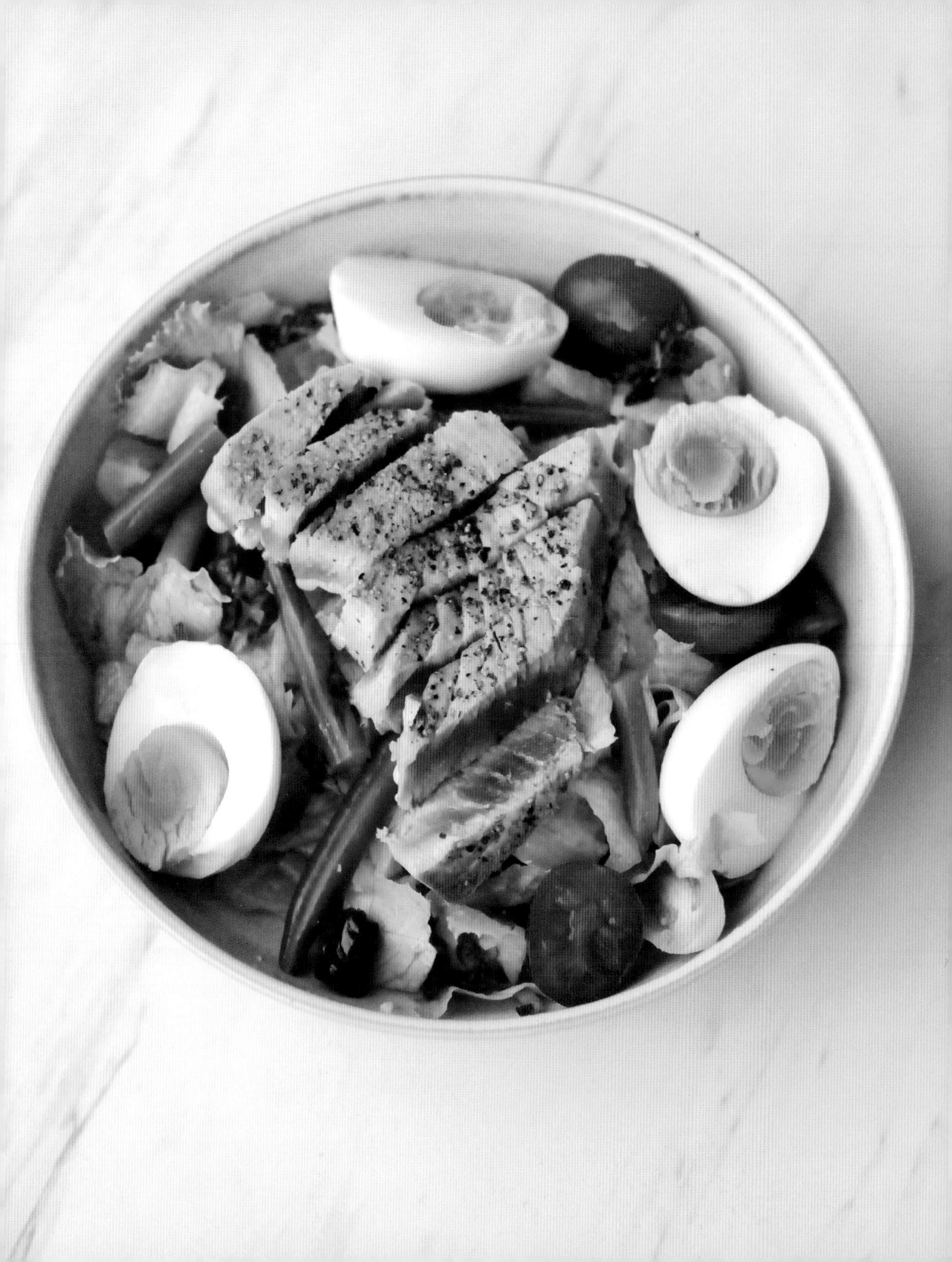

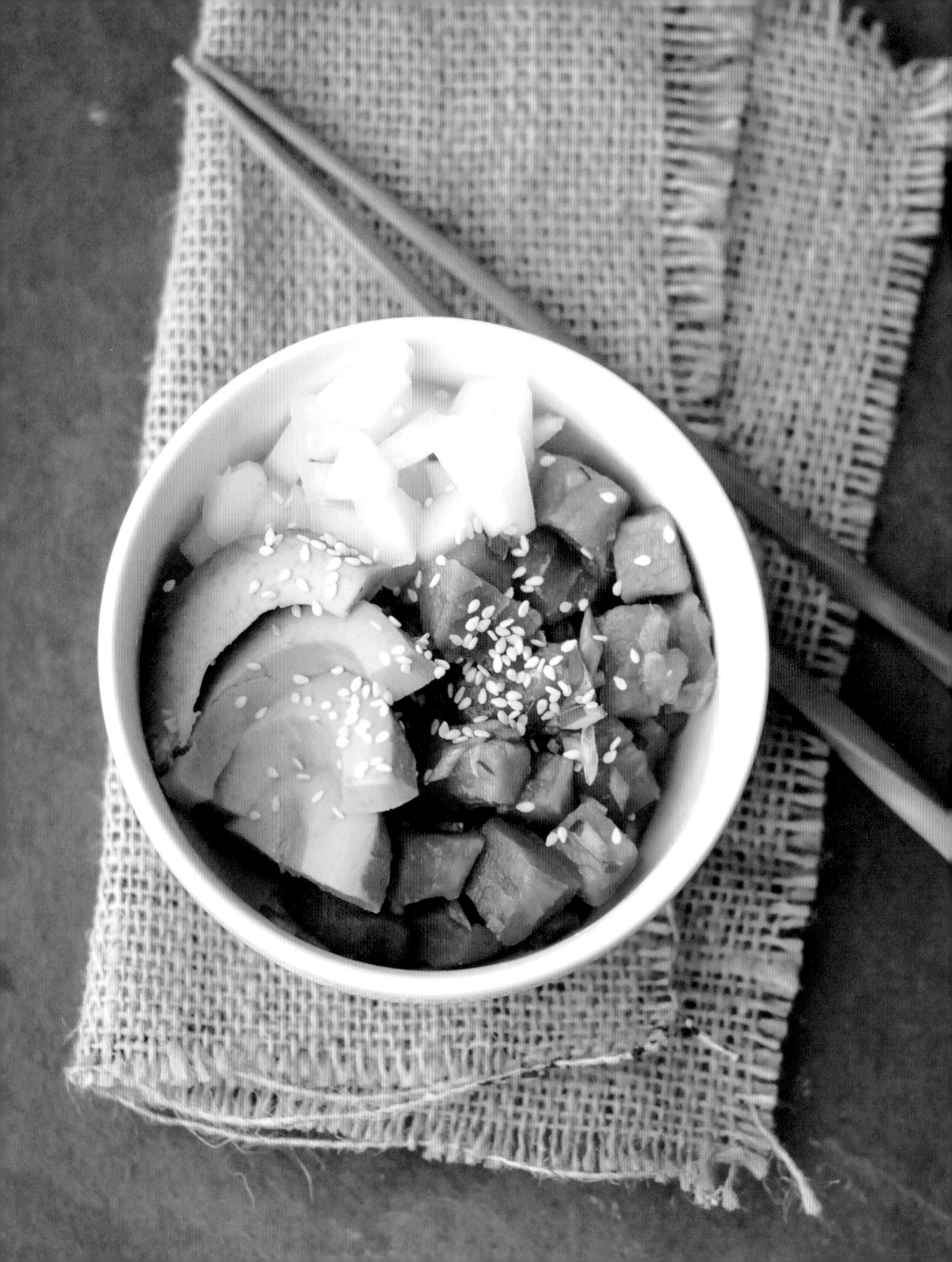

Poke Bowls with Avocado and Sesame Seeds DF NF

My friend Toyo and I love to surf together, and she lived in Hawaii for many years, so I learned to love poke from her. Make sure to use sushi- or sashimi-grade tuna when making this raw preparation.

YIELD: 4 servings | **PREP TIME:** 10 minutes | **COOK TIME:** 0 minutes

1 pound sashimi-grade ahi tuna, cut into ½-inch cubes

1 large shallot, minced

2 green onions, white and green parts, thinly sliced

¼ cup low-sodium soy sauce

2 tablespoons mirin

1 tablespoon toasted sesame oil

1 teaspoon sambal oelek chili paste

1 tablespoon sesame seeds

1 avocado, sliced

½ cucumber, peeled and diced

1. Place the tuna, shallot, and onions in a bowl.
2. In a separate container, whisk the soy sauce, mirin, sesame oil, and sambal oelek. Pour this over the tuna and toss gently to mix.
3. Divide the poke between serving bowls and top with the sesame seeds, avocado, and cucumber.

NUTRITION PER SERVING

CALORIES: 240 TOTAL FAT: 13g PROTEIN: 26g CARBOHYDRATES: 10g FIBER: 4g NET CARBS: 6g

Paella with Cauli Rice GF NF

There's a trick to getting paella right and it's even trickier with cauliflower rice—cook it too long, and you end up with mush. The secret is cooking the seafood and cauliflower separately and then serving them together. No, it's not real paella, but it still has all of the tasty flavors of seared chorizo, onion, garlic, tomatoes, and saffron infusing clams and shrimp with flavor.

YIELD: 4 servings | **PREP TIME:** 5 minutes | **COOK TIME:** 18 minutes

- 4 ounces chorizo sausage
- ½ cup minced yellow onion
- 2 teaspoons minced garlic
- 1 plum tomato, diced
- 1 tablespoon minced fresh oregano (1 teaspoon dried)
- 1 generous pinch of saffron, placed in 1 tablespoon warm water to steep
- 1 teaspoon smoked paprika
- 1 pound live clams, scrubbed
- 1 pound shrimp, peeled and deveined
- 1 recipe Cauli Rice (page 100)
- lemon wedges
- fresh parsley

1. Heat a large skillet over medium-high heat. When it's hot, add the chorizo, breaking it up with a wooden spoon. Cook for 2 to 3 minutes.
2. Add the onion and garlic and cook for 5 minutes, until the onion is soft. Add the tomato and oregano. Cook for 1 minute. Add the saffron "tea" and smoked paprika.
3. Add the clams to the pan and cover with a lid. Steam for 5 minutes. Add the shrimp to the pan and steam for another 5 minutes, until the seafood is cooked through.
4. Divide the Cauli Rice between serving bowls and top with the seafood mixture. Garnish with lemon and fresh parsley.

NUTRITION PER SERVING

CALORIES: 393 **TOTAL FAT:** 23g **PROTEIN:** 35g **CARBOHYDRATES:** 12g **FIBER:** 5g **NET CARBS:** 7g

Spicy Mussels with Roasted Fennel and Tomatoes DF GF NF

This dish is a harmonious blend of spicy, succulent mussels and redolent roasted tomatoes and fennel. Serve as a hearty dinner with a side of grain-free bread.

YIELD: 4 servings | **PREP TIME:** 10 minutes | **COOK TIME:** 30 minutes

- 4 plum tomatoes, halved
- 1 fennel bulb, cut into 8 wedges
- 6 tablespoons extra-virgin olive oil, divided
- ½ red onion, thinly sliced vertically
- 2 garlic cloves, smashed
- ¼ teaspoon red chili flakes
- 1 teaspoon fennel seeds, roughly ground in a mortar and pestle
- 1½ pounds mussels, scrubbed and debearded
- ½ cup chicken stock
- ½ cup dry white wine
- ¼ cup roughly chopped flat-leaf parsley
- sea salt
- freshly ground pepper

1. Preheat the oven to 325°F. Place the tomatoes in a bowl and drizzle with 2 tablespoons of the oil. Toss gently to coat in the oil. Spread the tomatoes out onto a baking sheet. Season with salt and pepper.
2. Repeat with the fennel. Toss in a bowl with 2 tablespoons olive oil, spread onto the baking sheet, and season with salt and pepper. Bake for 30 minutes, flipping the fennel about halfway through. The tomatoes should be juicy and beginning to brown. The fennel should be very tender and gently browned.
3. Meanwhile, place a large pot over medium-high heat with the remaining 2 tablespoons of oil. Add the red onion and cook for 5 minutes or until nearly soft.
4. Add the garlic, red chili flakes, and fennel to the pot and cook for 30 seconds, just until fragrant. Add the chicken stock and white wine and then add the mussels. Stir and then cover the pot with a lid. Reduce the heat to medium. Steam for 8 minutes, or until the mussels have all opened. Discard any that haven't opened at 10 minutes.
5. To serve, divide the roasted tomatoes and fennel between serving dishes. Top with the mussels and season generously with fresh parsley.

NUTRITION PER SERVING

CALORIES: 392 **TOTAL FAT:** 28g **PROTEIN:** 23g **CARBOHYDRATES:** 11g **FIBER:** 3g **NET CARBS:** 8g

Grilled Swordfish with Caper Gremolata DF GF NF

Piquant anchovy caper gremolata is the perfect complement to grilled swordfish and plum tomatoes with blanched green beans.

YIELD: 4 servings | **PREP TIME:** 10 minutes | **COOK TIME:** 15 minutes

3 tablespoons balsamic vinegar
3 tablespoons capers, rinsed and drained
4 anchovy fillets, roughly chopped
2 cloves garlic, minced
½ cup flat-leaf parsley
¼ cup plus 1 tablespoon extra-virgin olive oil
8 ounces green beans
4 (4- to 6-ounce) swordfish steaks
4 plum tomatoes, halved
sea salt
freshly ground pepper

1. To make the gremolata, combine the vinegar, capers, anchovies, garlic, parsley, and ¼ cup of olive oil in a blender or food processor. I like to use the cup that comes with my immersion blender. Blend until mostly smooth but still somewhat textured. Set aside.
2. Bring a large pot of salted water to a boil. Add the green beans and cook for 3 to 4 minutes, or until bright green and tender. Drain and set aside.
3. Heat a grill or grill pan to medium-high heat. Pat the swordfish dry with paper towels. Generously coat the swordfish and tomatoes with the remaining tablespoon of olive oil. Season the fish generously with salt and pepper.
4. Grill the fish for about 3 to 4 minutes on each side, until gently browned and beginning to feel firm to the touch. Grill the tomatoes cut-side down for 7 minutes.
5. To assemble the bowls, divide the green beans and grilled tomatoes between serving bowls. Top with the grilled swordfish and a generous spoonful of the gremolata.

COOKING TIP: Use the best-quality balsamic vinegar you can find. It should be thick and syrupy. A balsamic reduction is a good option, but don't use balsamic glaze, which usually has added sugar, among other questionable ingredients.

NUTRITION PER SERVING

CALORIES: 388 TOTAL FAT: 24g PROTEIN: 35g CARBOHYDRATES: 7g FIBER: 3g NET CARBS: 4g

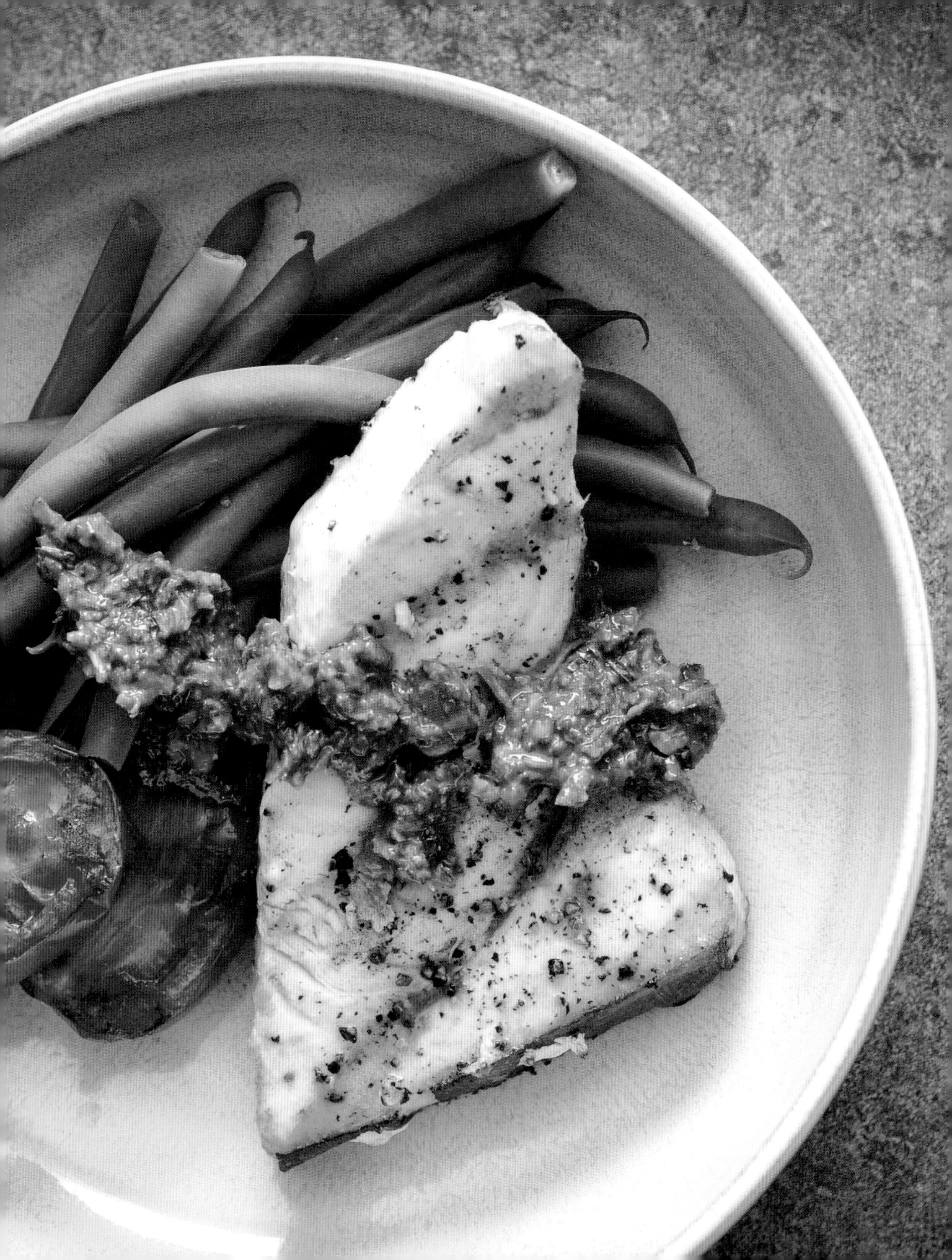

CHAPTER FIVE

BEEF & LAMB

Every culture has its standout red meat recipes—beef bourguignon in France, steak fajitas in Mexico, and lamb curry in India. I tried to visit several corners of the globe in this chapter to bring you a diversity of flavors and textures. Some bowls are fit for a light lunch—try the Skirt Steak with Herb Salad, Peanuts, and Cucumber Noodles. Others are perfect for a comforting dinner, like the Spaghetti Squash Marinara. I hope every one makes it into your recipe rotation.

- Spaghetti Squash Marinara
- Steak Fajita Bowls
- Meatballs over Mashed Cauliflower
- Beef Bourguignon over Mashed Cauliflower
- Skirt Steak with Herb Salad, Peanuts, and Cucumber Noodles
- Lamb Kebabs with Red Pepper–Cucumber Salad and Yogurt Sauce
- Lamb Curry over Cauli Rice with Cilantro Salsa

Spaghetti Squash Marinara DF GF NF

Until recently, I've been willing to spend a long time in the kitchen preparing a meal. As a cookbook author, it has been part of my job, after all. However, I recently accepted a position as an editor at a tech company. Gone are the leisurely afternoons letting a pot of marinara sauce simmer on the stove or carefully chopping lots of vegetables from the farmers market. Nevertheless, I still care about getting a healthy meal on the table. I'm guessing you feel the same. This recipe is easy-peasy with jarred marinara sauce and roasted spaghetti squash that takes only a few more minutes than boiling water for pasta.

YIELD: 4 servings | **PREP TIME:** 5 minutes | **COOK TIME:** 5 minutes (plus 30 minutes for cooking spaghetti squash)

- 1 pound ground beef
- 2 cups no-added-sugar marinara sauce
- 1 recipe Spaghetti Squash (page 102)
- 2 ounces (about ½ cup) grated Parmesan (optional)
- 4 fresh basil leaves, thinly sliced

1. In a large skillet, brown the ground beef for 2 to 3 minutes. Add the marinara sauce and simmer for another 2 to 3 minutes.
2. Divide the cooked spaghetti squash between serving bowls. Top with the beef and marinara sauce. Top with the Parmesan, if using, and the basil.

NUTRITION PER SERVING

CALORIES: 494 TOTAL FAT: 37g PROTEIN: 26g CARBOHYDRATES: 14g FIBER: 3g NET CARBS: 11g

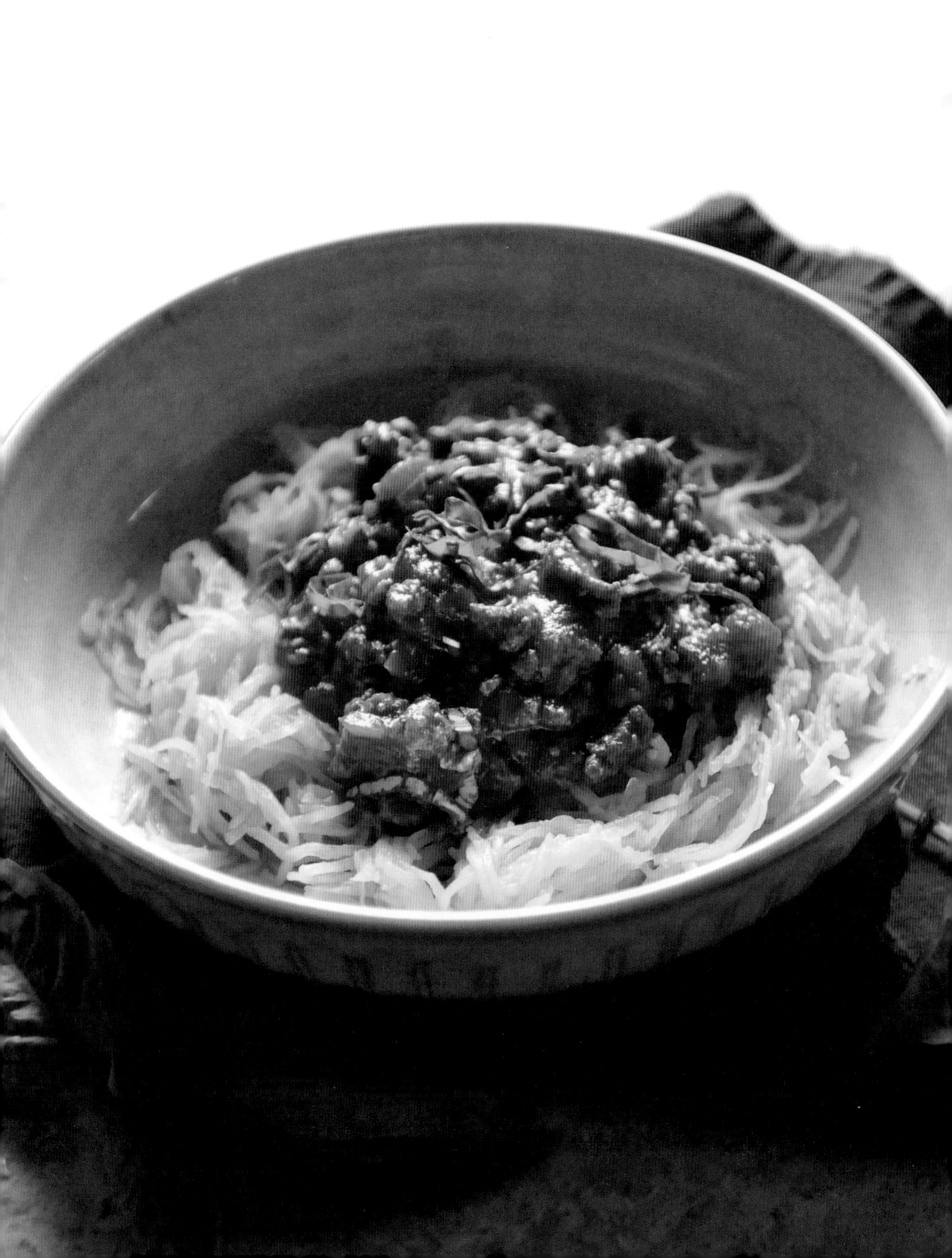

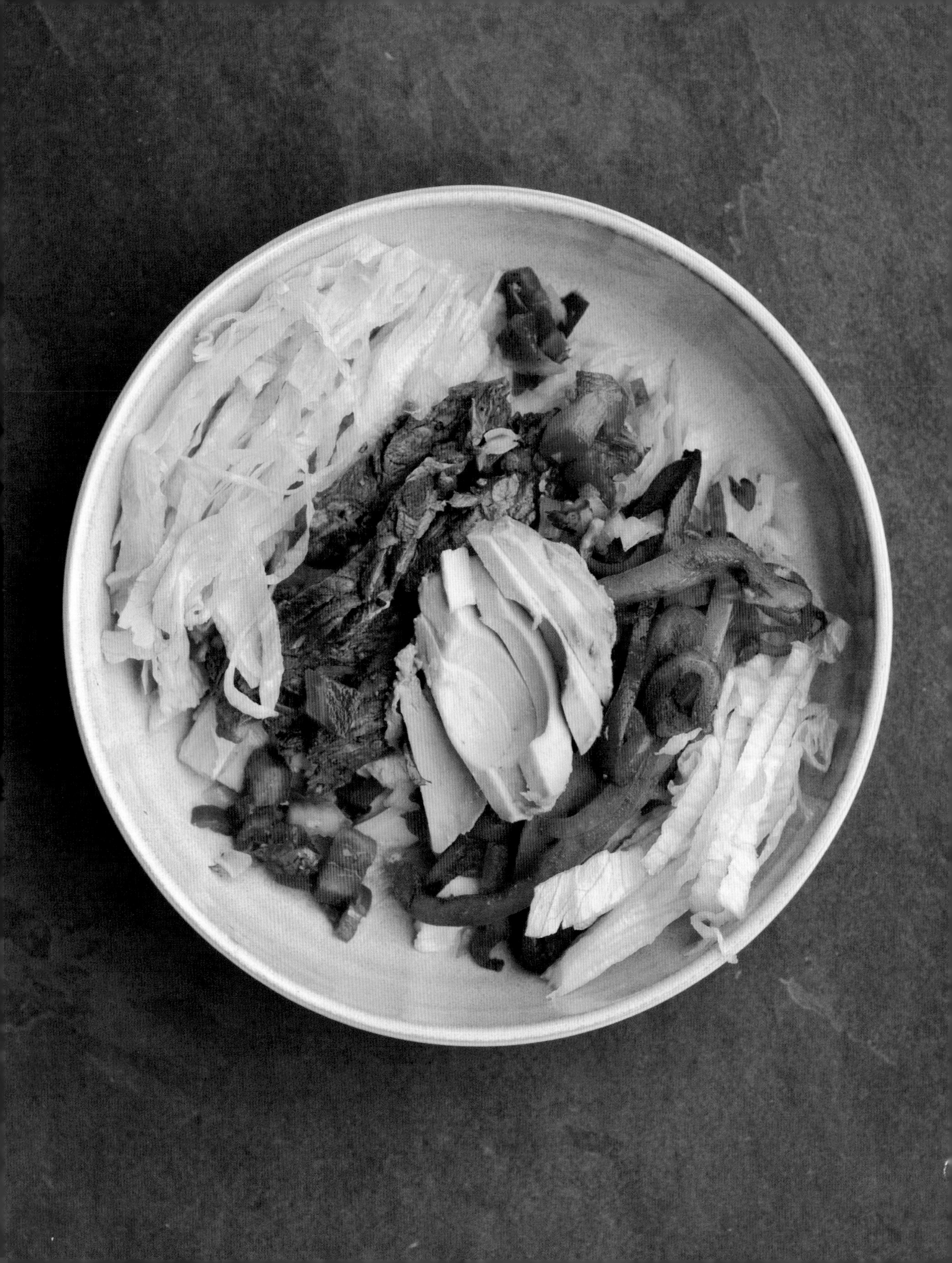

Steak Fajita Bowls DF GF NF

One of my closest friends is from Mexico and shared her method for making flank steak tacos with me. They're best done on an outdoor grill, but when we first made them together, the weather was cold (by California standards) and I didn't really feel like cooking outside. Instead, we used a cast-iron skillet, which worked beautifully and inspired me to make fajita bowls from the same recipe.

YIELD: 4 servings | **PREP TIME:** 5 minutes | **COOK TIME:** 10 minutes

- 1½ pounds flank steak
- 3 teaspoons extra-virgin olive oil, divided
- 1 tablespoon ancho chile powder
- 1 teaspoon smoked paprika
- kosher salt
- 2 bell peppers, any colors, cored, thinly sliced
- 1 yellow onion, thinly sliced
- 2 cups shredded lettuce
- 1 cup Guacamole (page 104) or store-bought guacamole
- ½ cup spicy salsa
- shredded lettuce, optional

1. Coat the steak in 1 teaspoon of the olive oil, chile powder, paprika, and a generous pinch of salt. Set aside.
2. Heat a cast-iron skillet over high heat. When it's hot, sear the flank steak for 2 minutes on each side, or until browned and nearly cooked through. Transfer to a cutting board to rest. You may have to do this in two batches if your steaks are very thin.
3. While the steak rests, add the remaining 2 teaspoons oil to the skillet and then add the peppers and onion. Sauté for 3 to 4 minutes. The vegetables will pick up some of the color from the spices used for the steak.
4. Slice the steak very thinly and divide between serving bowls. Add the vegetables and lettuce. Top with the guacamole and salsa. Garnish with shredded lettuce, if desired.

COOKING TIP: The best salsa for this recipe is salsa morita with tomatillos. A salsa verde is a good substitute, but it lacks the smoky quality of the morita chiles.

NUTRITION PER SERVING

CALORIES: 479 TOTAL FAT: 30g PROTEIN: 38g CARBOHYDRATES: 14g FIBER: 5g NET CARBS: 9g

Meatballs over Mashed Cauliflower GF

When you're feeling like comfort food, this bowl hits the spot. Creamy cauliflower forms a luxurious base. Top it off with hearty meatballs and a shower of fresh parsley. Most recipes in this book serve 4 or fewer. This one serves 6 because it has so many calories. That said, I've provided nutrition information for both serving sizes if you're feeling hungry.

YIELD: 6 (2-meatball) servings | **PREP TIME:** 10 minutes | **COOK TIME:** 30 to 37 minutes

1 tablespoon olive oil

1 small yellow onion, minced

4 cloves garlic, minced

12 ounces ground beef

12 ounces ground pork

½ cup tomato puree

½ cup almond meal

1 egg, whisked

1 teaspoon apple cider vinegar

1 tablespoon Italian herb blend

1 teaspoon sea salt

1 recipe Mashed Cauliflower (page 98)

¼ cup minced fresh parsley

1. Preheat the oven to 350°F. Line a sheet pan with parchment paper.
2. Heat the olive oil in a small skillet over medium heat. Cook the onion for 5 to 7 minutes, until softened. Add the garlic and cook for another minute. Remove the pan from the heat.
3. Combine the beef, pork, tomato puree, almond meal, egg, vinegar, herb blend, salt, and the cooked onion mixture. Mix gently with your hands until well combined. Do not overmix.
4. Divide the mixture into 12 portions and place them onto a sheet pan. Bake for 25 to 30 minutes, or until just cooked through.
5. Divide the Mashed Cauliflower between serving bowls and top with the meatballs and fresh parsley. Drizzle with additional tomato puree if desired.

COOKING TIP: For easy cooking and cleanup, place the meatball mixture into a muffin tin.

NUTRITION PER SERVING FOR 6 (2 MEATBALLS EACH)

CALORIES: 512 TOTAL FAT: 40g PROTEIN: 29g CARBOHYDRATES: 11g FIBER: 4g NET CARBS: 7g

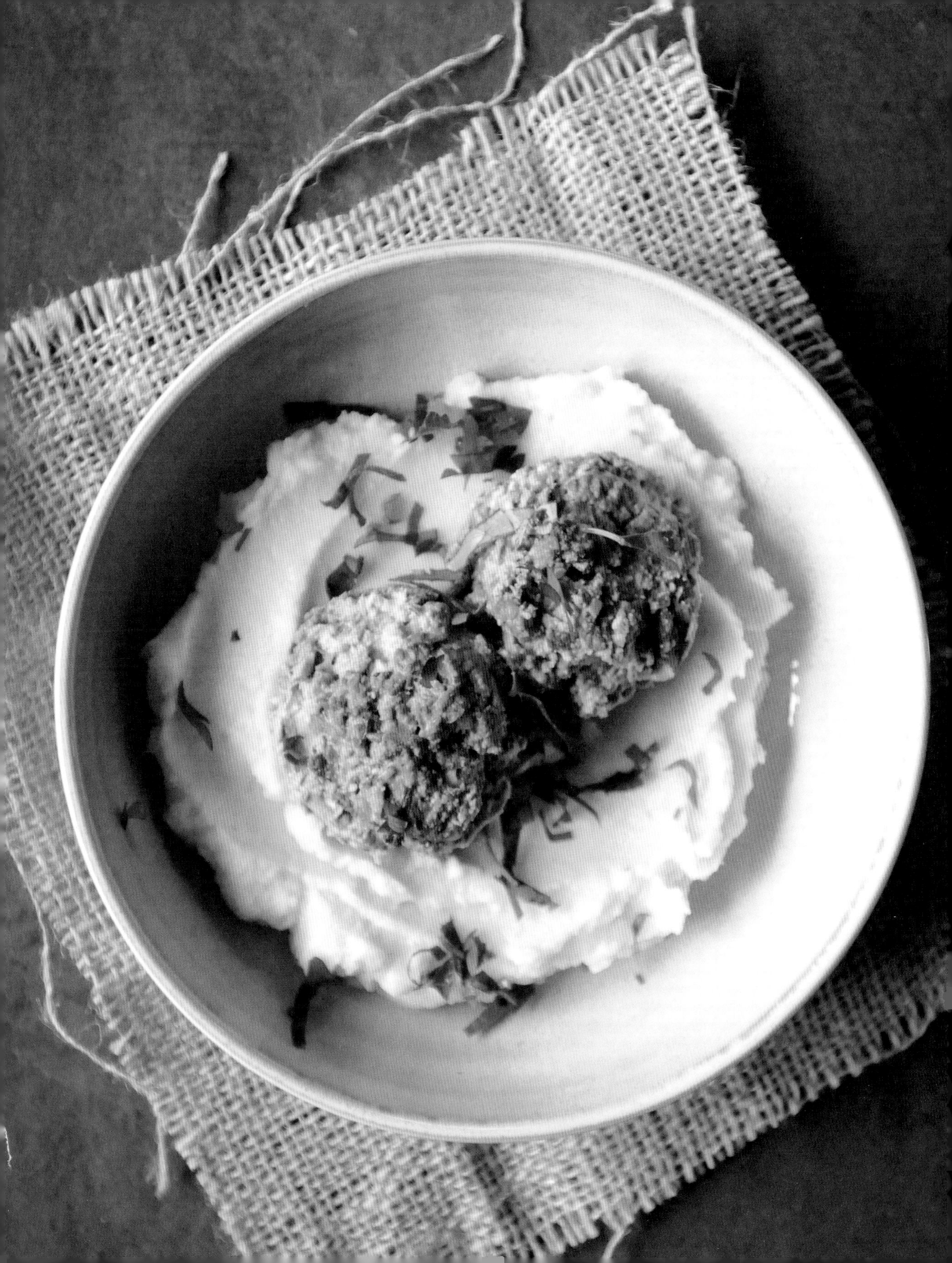

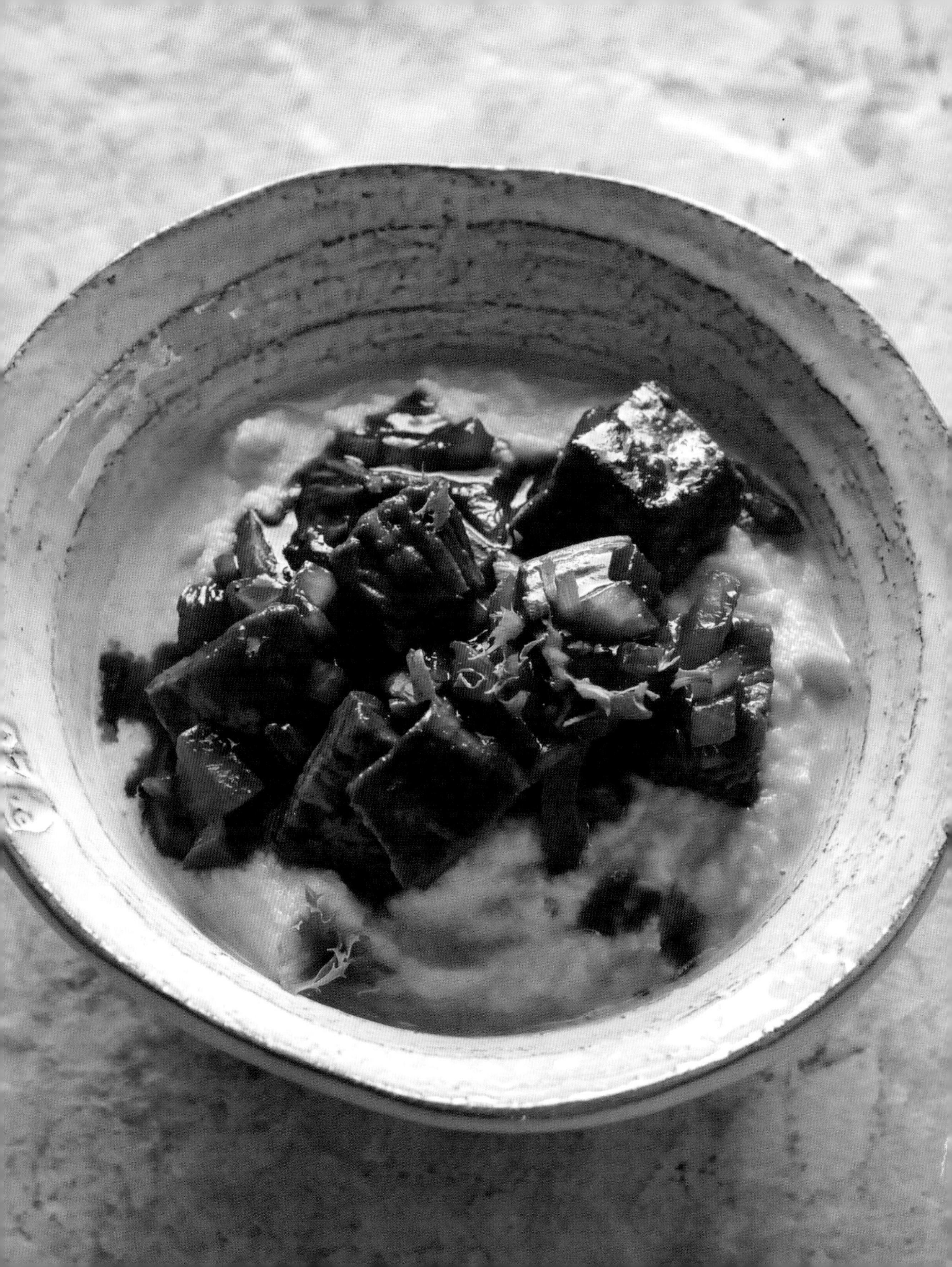

Beef Bourguignon over Mashed Cauliflower GF NF

Beef bourguignon was one of the first French dishes I learned to cook. The magic of long, slow braises is that they turn otherwise tough cuts of meat into tender, succulent dishes that feel opulent. It's one of the most essential techniques for good cooking and it is useful in your low-carb kitchen.

YIELD: 4 servings | **PREP TIME:** 10 minutes | **COOK TIME:** 3 hours 20 minutes

2 pounds beef chuck, cut into 2-inch cubes

kosher salt

freshly ground pepper

2 tablespoons canola oil

1 tablespoon tomato paste

2 cups dry red wine

2 cups low-sodium beef broth

8 ounces frozen pearl onions

1 sprig thyme

1 sprig rosemary

1 recipe Mashed Cauliflower (page 98)

2 tablespoons minced fresh parsley, for serving, optional

1. Heat a large pot over medium-high heat. Pat the beef cubes dry with paper towels and then season generously with salt and pepper.
2. Add the oil to the pot. When it's hot, place some of the beef into the pan, being careful not to crowd the pan. Sear until gently browned on all sides. You will need to sear the beef in batches. This will take 10 to 20 minutes. Remove the seared beef from the pan and set aside.
3. Add the tomato paste to the pan and cook for 1 to 2 minutes, until it begins to caramelize. Deglaze the pan with the wine, scraping up the browned bits from the bottom of the pan. Add the beef broth, pearl onions, thyme, and rosemary, and return the beef and any accumulated juices to the pot. Bring to a gentle simmer, cover, and cook over low heat for roughly three hours.
4. To serve, divide the Mashed Cauliflower between four bowls. Top with the beef bourguignon, garnish with fresh parsley, if using, and serve.

COOKING TIP: To make this go more quickly, use an Instant Pot to cook the beef bourguignon—it will take less than 1 hour, including searing the beef.

NUTRITION PER SERVING

CALORIES: 638 TOTAL FAT: 30g PROTEIN: 51g CARBOHYDRATES: 16g FIBER: 5g NET CARBS: 11g

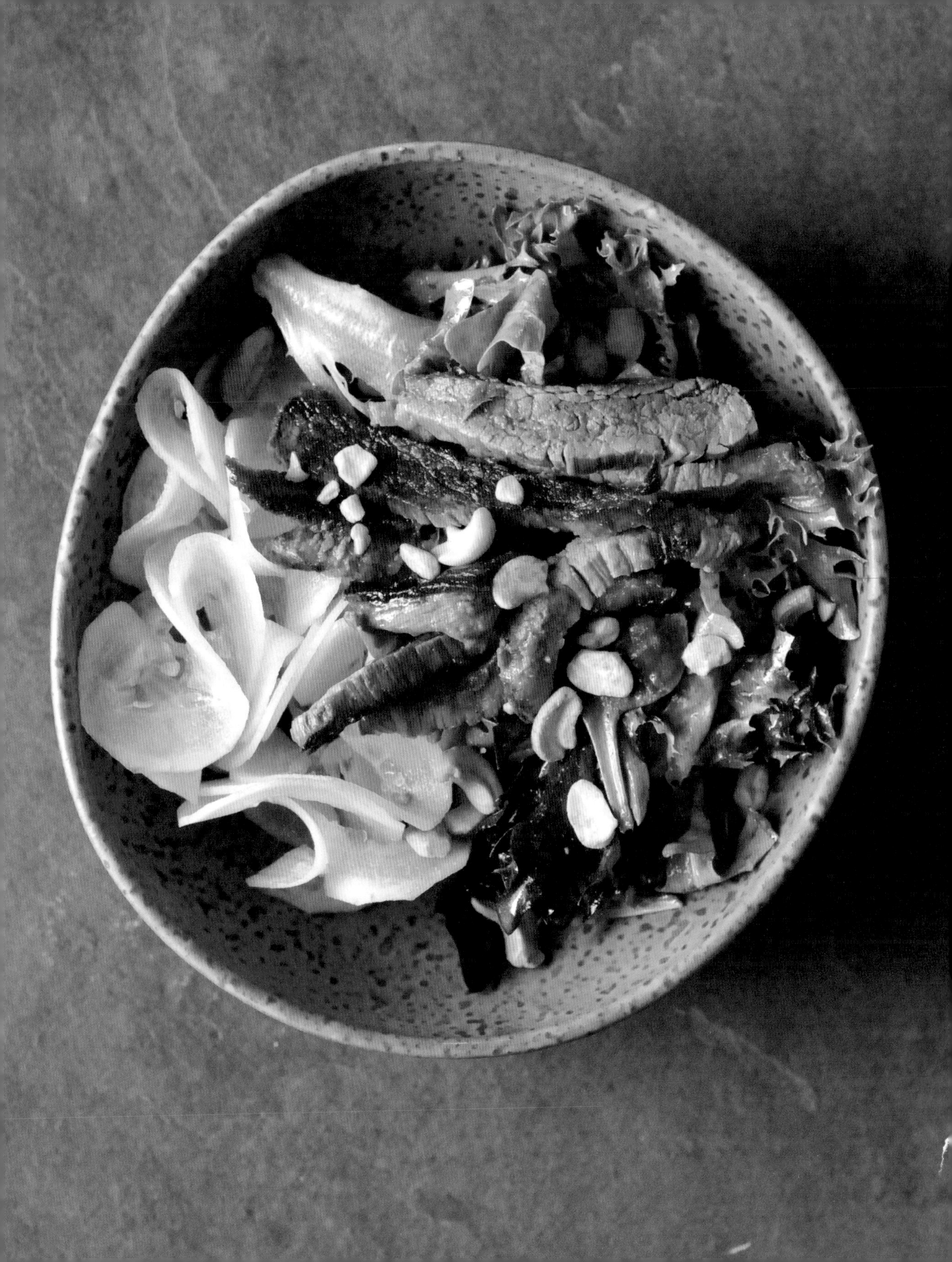

Skirt Steak with Herb Salad, Peanuts, and Cucumber Noodles DF

This salad is bursting with flavors of Southeast Asia. It's a little more work than takeout, but it's worth it!

YIELD: 4 servings | **PREP TIME:** 10 minutes | **COOK TIME:** 5 minutes

FOR THE STEAK:

1 tablespoon toasted sesame oil

1 tablespoon lime juice

2 tablespoons soy sauce

¼ teaspoon cayenne pepper

1 pound skirt steak

FOR THE HERB SALAD:

1 medium cucumber, peeled

1 shallot, minced

1 tablespoon lime juice

1 teaspoon minced ginger

1 small clove garlic, minced

3 tablespoons extra-virgin olive oil

1 drop liquid stevia, optional

½ cup roughly chopped basil

½ cup roughly chopped cilantro

2 cups baby lettuces

¼ cup finely chopped roasted peanuts

1. To make the steak, whisk the sesame oil, lime juice, soy sauce, and cayenne in a shallow dish. Add the skirt steak and turn to coat in the mixture. This can be done up to a day ahead of time. Set aside to marinate for at least 10 minutes.
2. Heat a grill or grill pan to medium-high heat. Remove the steak from the marinade and sear for 2 to 3 minutes on each side, depending on the thickness of the steak. Set on a cutting board to rest for 5 minutes, then slice thinly on a bias.
3. To make the cucumber noodles, fit your spiralizer with the wide slicing blade. Spiralize according to the instructions for Vegetable Noodles on page 103.
4. To make the herb salad, whisk the shallot, lime juice, ginger, garlic, and olive oil in a small bowl. Add a drop of liquid stevia if you like. Just before serving, add the basil, cilantro, and lettuce to the bowl and toss very gently to coat the leaves in the dressing.
5. To serve, divide the cucumber noodles and herb salad between serving bowls. Top with the steak and garnish with peanuts.

NUTRITION PER SERVING

CALORIES: 396 TOTAL FAT: 30g PROTEIN: 27g CARBOHYDRATES: 5g FIBER: 2g NET CARBS: 3g

Lamb Kebabs with Red Pepper–Cucumber Salad and Yogurt Sauce GF NF

Spicy cayenne and black peppers and fragrant cinnamon permeate these lamb kebabs. They're served with a crunchy salad of red bell peppers and cucumber with a cooling garlic yogurt sauce on the side. They're tasty as a bowl or yummy stuffed into a low-carb coconut wrap. They're also perfect for meal prepping—just keep the yogurt sauce on the side.

YIELD: 4 servings | **PREP TIME:** 10 minutes | **COOK TIME:** 8 minutes

FOR THE LAMB KEBABS:

½ teaspoon cayenne pepper

⅛ teaspoon ground cinnamon

1 teaspoon dried mint

1 teaspoon minced garlic

1 teaspoon sea salt

1 teaspoon ground black pepper

2 tablespoons extra-virgin olive oil, divided

1½ pounds lamb loin, trimmed and cut into 1-inch pieces

FOR THE RED PEPPER–CUCUMBER SALAD:

1 cucumber, diced

1 red bell pepper, cored and diced

½ jalapeno pepper, minced

½ cup roughly chopped fresh mint leaves

1 tablespoon minced fresh dill

1 tablespoon extra-virgin olive oil

1 teaspoon lemon juice

sea salt

freshly ground pepper

FOR THE YOGURT SAUCE:

½ cup whole-milk, plain yogurt

1 teaspoon minced garlic

1 tablespoon lemon juice

¼ teaspoon sea salt

1. To make the lamb kebabs, combine the cayenne pepper, cinnamon, mint, garlic, salt, pepper, and olive oil in a shallow dish. Place the lamb shoulder into the mixture and turn to coat it in the spices. Set aside to marinate for up to one day.
2. Remove the lamb from the marinade and thread onto metal or bamboo skewers.
3. Heat a grill or grill pan to medium-high heat. Cook the lamb for 3 to 4 minutes on each side, or until cooked through to your desired level of doneness.

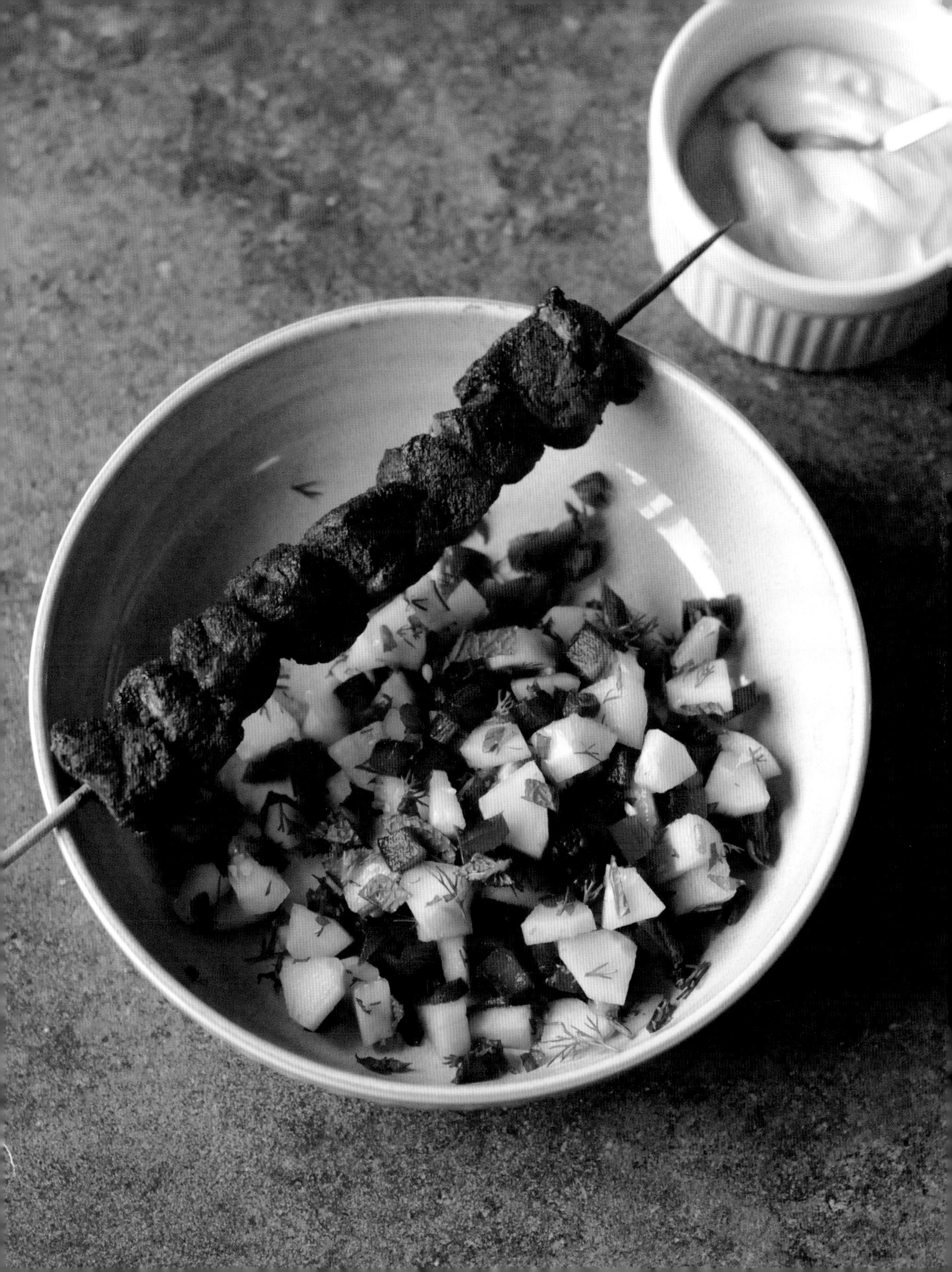

4. To make the red pepper–cucumber salad, combine the cucumber, bell pepper, jalapeno pepper, mint, and dill in a bowl. Drizzle with the olive oil and lemon juice and season to taste with salt and pepper.
5. To make the yogurt sauce, whisk the yogurt, garlic, lemon juice, and salt in a small bowl.
6. To serve, divide the red pepper–cucumber salad between shallow serving bowls. Top with the lamb kebabs and drizzle with yogurt sauce.

COOKING TIP: If you prefer the taste of beef, or it's more accessible, feel free to use it in place of the lamb. Choose a tender cut of steak such as sirloin.

NUTRITION PER SERVING

CALORIES: 470 TOTAL FAT: 25g PROTEIN: 54g CARBOHYDRATES: 6g FIBER: 1g NET CARBS: 5g

Lamb Curry over Cauli Rice with Cilantro Salsa GF NF

This spicy Indian curry gets its flavor from ginger, garlic, cayenne pepper, and a bevy of Indian spices. It's balanced with a crunchy onion and cilantro salsa and a refreshing yogurt sauce and served over a bed of Cauli Rice. It takes a little time to prepare, so plan to make it on the weekend when you can let things simmer away on the stove. Enjoy with a glass of Riesling or another crisp white wine.

YIELD: 4 servings | **PREP TIME:** 10 minutes | **COOK TIME:** 2½ to 3 hours

FOR THE LAMB CURRY:

1 teaspoon ground turmeric

½ teaspoon ground cumin

½ teaspoon ground coriander

⅛ teaspoon cayenne pepper

1 teaspoon ground black pepper

1½ pounds lamb shoulder

2 tablespoons canola oil

1 teaspoon minced fresh ginger

1 teaspoon minced fresh garlic

½ red onion, thinly sliced

FOR THE CILANTRO SALSA:

1 cup minced cilantro

½ red onion, minced

2 green onions, white and green parts, thinly sliced

½ teaspoon sea salt

2 tablespoons lemon juice

FOR THE YOGURT SAUCE:

½ cup whole-milk, plain yogurt

1 teaspoon minced garlic

1 tablespoon lemon juice

¼ teaspoon sea salt

1 recipe Cauli Rice (page 100)

1. Combine the turmeric, cumin, coriander, cayenne pepper, and black pepper in a shallow dish. Add the lamb shoulder and turn gently to coat it in the spice mixture.
2. Heat the canola oil in a large pot over medium-high heat. Sear the lamb until it is well browned on all sides. Add the ginger, garlic, and onion. Cook for 30 seconds, just until fragrant.
3. Add 2 cups of water and bring to a simmer. Cover and reduce the heat to low. Cook for 2½ to 3 hours, or until the lamb is tender.

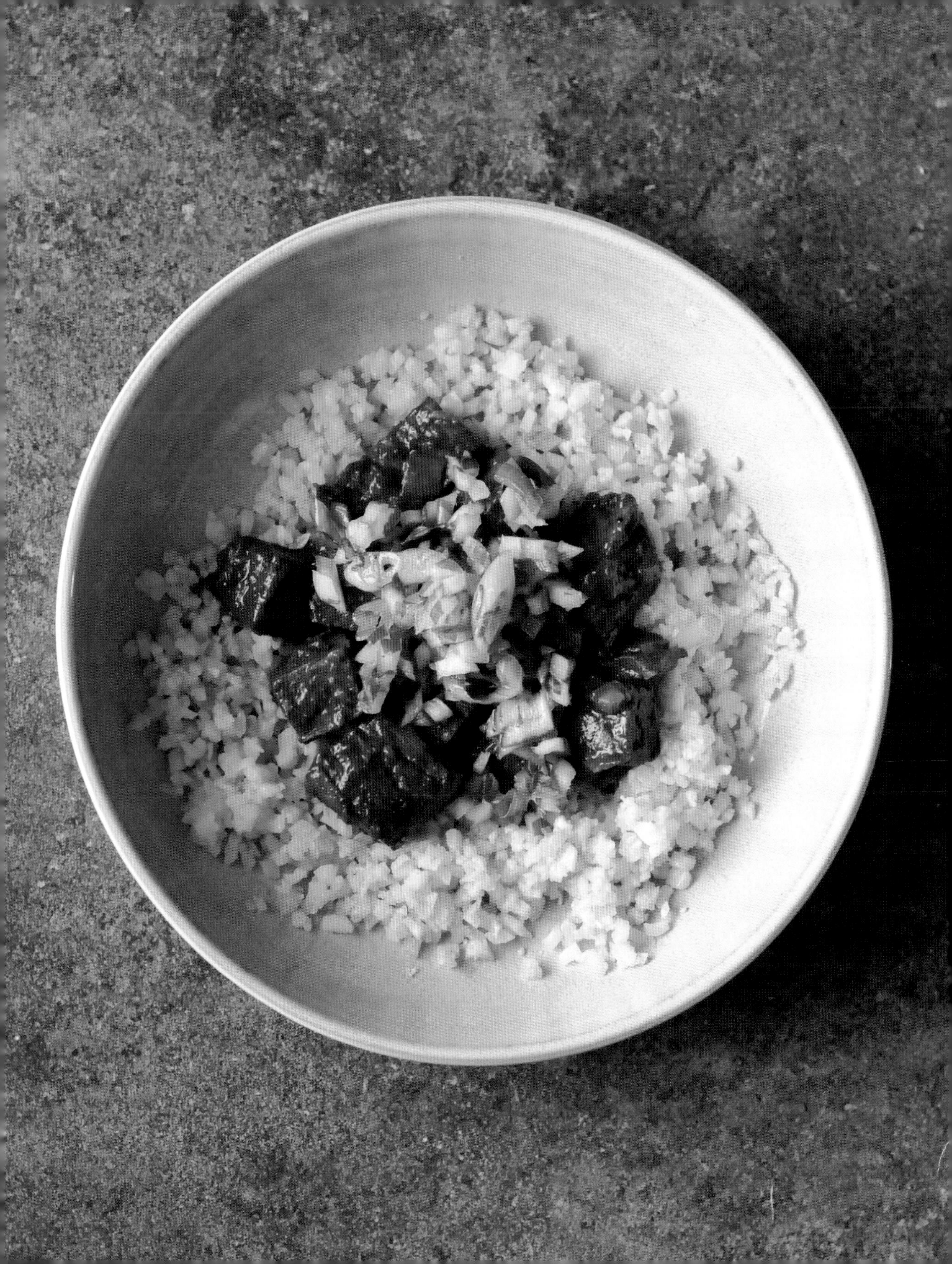

4. To make the cilantro salsa, combine the cilantro, red onion, green onion, salt, and lemon juice in a small, nonreactive dish. Refrigerate until ready to serve.
5. To make the yogurt sauce, whisk together the yogurt, garlic, lemon juice, and salt. Refrigerate until ready to serve.
6. To serve, divide the Cauli Rice between serving dishes. Top with the lamb curry, cilantro salsa, and yogurt sauce.

COOKING TIP: To make this dish in under an hour, make it in an Instant Pot.

NUTRITION PER SERVING

CALORIES: 508 TOTAL FAT: 26g PROTEIN: 57g CARBOHYDRATES: 13g FIBER: 5g NET CARBS: 7g

CHAPTER SIX

PORK

Have you noticed that you only need a little pork to liven up just about any dish? The juicy meat is loaded with flavor. Go bold with the Chorizo, Bell Peppers, and Cauli Rice with Salsa Verde for a festive meal. For something a little more refined, opt for the Roasted Pork Tenderloin with Cabbage Slaw over Mashed Cauliflower.

- Guajillo Braised Pork Taco Bowls
- Asian Meatball Noodle Bowls
- Chorizo, Bell Peppers, and Cauli Rice with Salsa Verde
- Sausage and Grilled Veggie Bowls
- Pork Chili Verde Bowls
- Roasted Pork Tenderloin with Cabbage Slaw over Mashed Cauliflower
- Pork Panzanella

Guajillo Braised Pork Taco Bowls DF GF NF

I prepared this recipe for a crowd of twenty at a surf retreat and it was a huge hit. The recipe is inspired by one in the book *Salt, Fat, Acid, Heat*. The original calls for beer, and I cut it with a bit of broth to keep the carbs in check. It's excellent for meal prepping and freezes beautifully.

YIELD: 4 servings | **PREP TIME:** 15 minutes | **COOK TIME:** 2½ to 3 hours

- 1 tablespoon coconut oil
- 1½ pounds pork shoulder (also called pork butt), cut into 1-inch cubes
- sea salt
- freshly ground pepper
- ½ yellow onion, quartered
- 8 cloves garlic, smashed and peeled
- 2 to 3 guajillo chiles
- 1 cup crushed tomatoes
- 1 tablespoon ground cumin
- 12 ounces light beer
- 1 to 2 cups chicken broth
- ½ red onion, thinly sliced
- 2 tablespoons red wine vinegar
- 4 cups shredded cabbage
- 1 avocado, sliced

1. Preheat the oven to 325°F.
2. Heat the coconut oil in a large Dutch oven over medium-high heat. Season the pork shoulder with salt and pepper and cook in the oil until well browned on all sides, about 10 minutes.
3. Add the onion, garlic, chiles, tomatoes, cumin, and beer. Add broth until the pork is just covered.
4. Place the lid on the pot and roast for 2½ to 3 hours, or until the pork is easily shredded with a fork.
5. While the pork is cooking, combine the red onion with the red wine vinegar and season with salt. Set aside to let the onions mellow.
6. To serve, divide the cabbage between serving bowls. Top with the braised pork, pickled onion, and a few slices of avocado.

COOKING TIP: The braised pork doubles easily. Make an extra batch and freeze leftovers.

NUTRITION PER SERVING

CALORIES: 713 TOTAL FAT: 51g PROTEIN: 43g CARBOHYDRATES: 14g FIBER: 6g NET CARBS: 7g

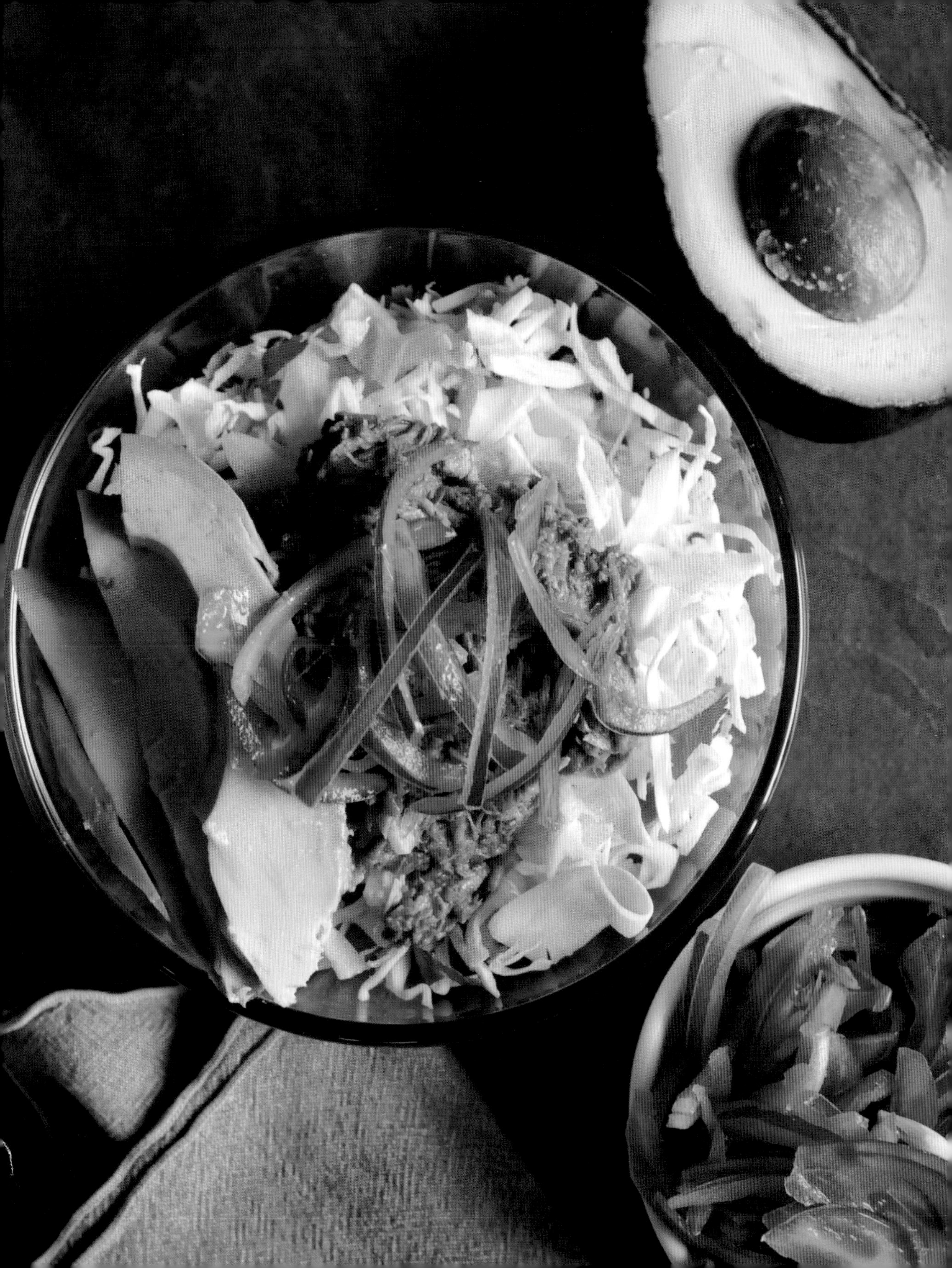

Asian Meatball Noodle Bowls DF NF

The Asian flavors in these pork meatballs make them a fun change of pace from the traditional Italian flavors of oregano and tomatoes. Serve them in lettuce cups, with Cauli Rice (page 100), or over zucchini noodles (page 103) with plenty of extra soy sauce and lime juice.

YIELD: 4 servings | **PREP TIME:** 10 minutes | **COOK TIME:** 15 minutes

- 1 egg, whisked
- ¼ cup almond flour
- 1 teaspoon minced ginger
- 1 teaspoon minced garlic
- ½ teaspoon sea salt
- ¼ teaspoon freshly ground pepper
- ¼ cup minced cilantro
- 1 cup roughly chopped spinach
- 1 green onion, white and green parts, thinly sliced
- 1 pound ground pork
- 2 tablespoons coconut oil
- ¼ cup soy sauce
- 2 tablespoons lime juice
- 1 teaspoon sambal oelek or another chili paste
- ¼ cup canola oil
- 1 recipe Spaghetti Squash (page 102)
- 1 cup shredded cabbage
- ¼ cup minced cilantro
- ¼ cup minced fresh mint
- 1 carrot, peeled, julienned

1. Combine the egg, almond flour, ginger, garlic, salt, and pepper in a large mixing bowl. Stir in the cilantro, spinach, and green onion.
2. Add the pork and use your hands to combine the mixture. Shape it into 8 to 12 balls.
3. Heat a large skillet over medium-high heat. Melt the coconut oil. When it's hot, sear the meatballs on all sides until well browned and cooked through, about 15 minutes total.
4. Whisk the soy sauce, lime juice, sambal oelek, and canola oil in a large bowl. Add the Spaghetti Squash and cabbage and toss gently to coat. Divide this between serving bowls.
5. Top with the cooked meatballs, cilantro, mint, and carrot.

NUTRITION PER SERVING

CALORIES: 630 FAT: 49g PROTEIN: 34g TOTAL CARBS: 13g FIBER: 4g NET CARBS: 9g

Chorizo, Bell Peppers, and Cauli Rice with Salsa Verde DF GF NF

Chorizo is spiced ground pork that brings so much flavor to any dish. Here, it's paired with sautéed bell peppers and onion and Cauli Rice and then drizzled with a punchy salsa verde sauce. It's great for meal prepping—just keep the salsa verde in a separate container until you heat up the chorizo and rice mixture.

YIELD: 4 servings | **PREP TIME:** 10 minutes | **COOK TIME:** 6 to 10 minutes

- 1 pound chorizo
- 1 red bell pepper, cored and sliced
- 1 green bell pepper, cored and sliced
- ½ yellow onion, sliced
- 1 recipe Cauli Rice (page 100)
- 1 recipe Salsa Verde (page 108)

1. Heat a large skillet over medium-high heat. Add the chorizo, breaking it up with a wooden spoon. Cook for 3 to 5 minutes, until it has rendered some of its fat.
2. Add the bell peppers and onion and sauté until the vegetables are crisp-tender, another 3 to 5 minutes.
3. Add the Cauli Rice to the pan and give everything a quick stir to incorporate. Divide this between serving plates and drizzle with the Salsa Verde.

NUTRITION PER SERVING

CALORIES: 460 TOTAL FAT: 36g PROTEIN: 21g CARBOHYDRATES: 16g FIBER: 7g NET CARBS: 9g

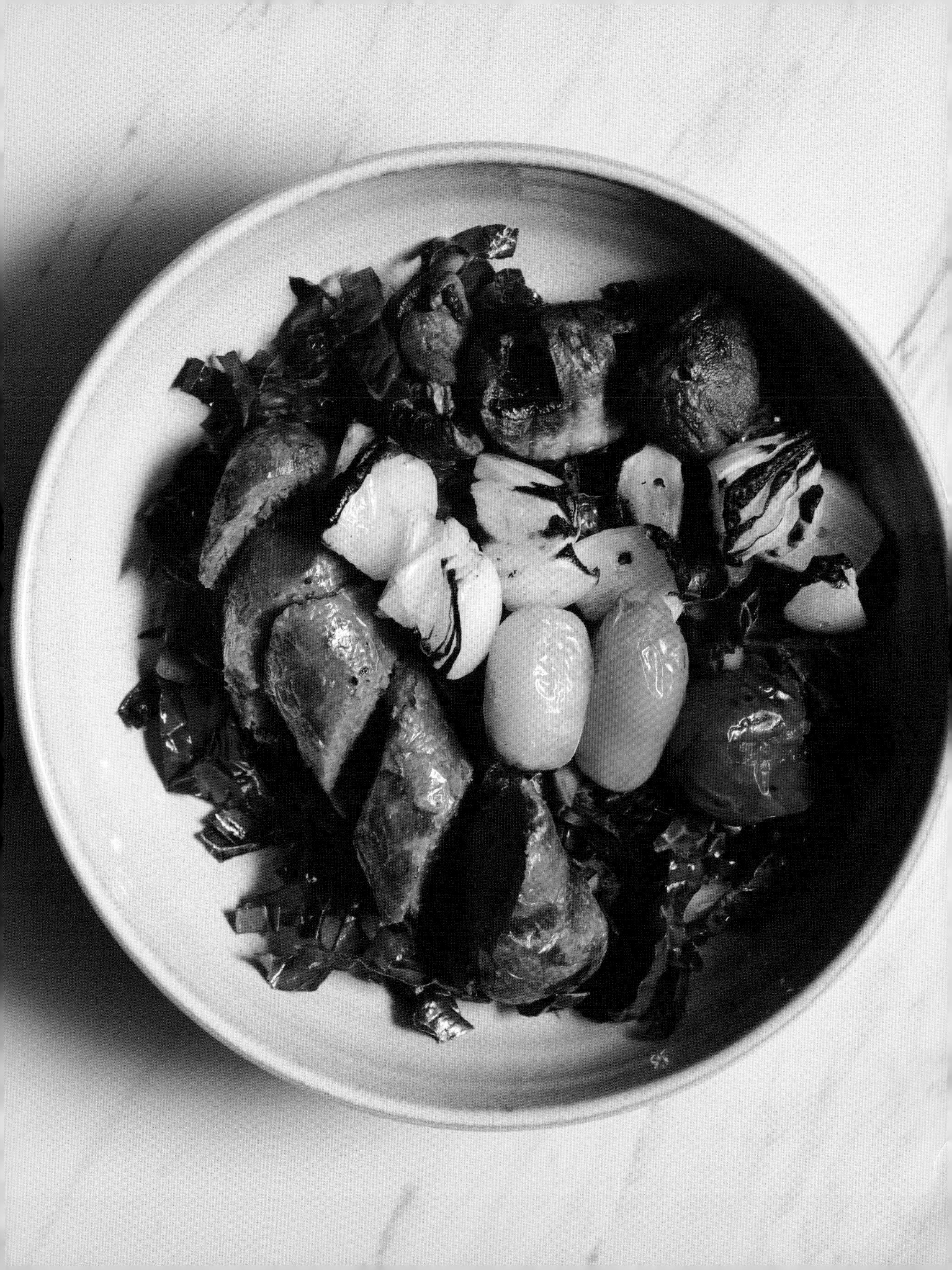

Sausage and Grilled Veggie Bowls DF GF NF

After cooking with charcoal for years, we finally bought a gas grill. Now I want to grill everything—it's so easy! This bowl came together in a flash of inspiration when the weather was warm and I had lots of vegetables in the kitchen that were begging to get used up.

YIELD: 4 servings | **PREP TIME:** 10 minutes | **COOK TIME:** 10 minutes

- 1 bunch kale, shredded
- 4 tablespoons extra-virgin olive oil, divided
- sea salt
- freshly ground pepper
- 1 teaspoon red wine vinegar
- 1 pint cremini mushrooms, halved
- 1 pint grape or cherry tomatoes
- 1 small yellow onion
- 4 (4-ounce) pork sausages, such as bratwurst

1. Place the kale in a bowl and drizzle with 1 tablespoon of the oil. Season with salt and pepper. Massage the kale until it is a deep green and soft, about 1 minute. Toss with the red wine vinegar.
2. Preheat a grill to medium-high heat. Thread the mushrooms, tomatoes, and onion onto individual skewers. Alternately, place them in a grill basket. Brush the vegetables with the remaining olive oil and season generously with salt and pepper.
3. Grill the vegetables and the sausages for 10 minutes, turning frequently until the vegetables are gently browned and soft and the sausage is cooked through.
4. Divide the kale between serving bowls and top with the sausage and vegetables.

NUTRITION PER SERVING

CALORIES: 518 FAT: 45g PROTEIN: 18g TOTAL CARBS: 12g FIBER: 3g NET CARBS: 9g

Pork Chili Verde Bowls GF NF

Use an Instant Pot to make this meal in a matter of minutes—okay, it takes 45 minutes, but not bad for a hearty stew! You can also make it in a Dutch oven, but it will take 2½ to 3 hours on the stovetop. Top with avocado, green onions, mozzarella cheese, and sour cream for a decadent meal.

YIELD: 4 servings | **PREP TIME:** 5 minutes | **COOK TIME:** 45 minutes

1 tablespoon canola oil

1 pound pork shoulder, cut into 1-inch cubes

1 yellow onion, halved and cut into thick slices

2 cloves garlic, smashed

1 (16-ounce jar) fire-roasted salsa verde

½ cup shredded mozzarella cheese

1 small avocado, pitted and thinly sliced

½ cup sour cream

2 green onions, white and green parts, thinly sliced

½ cup minced cilantro

sea salt

freshly ground pepper

1. Preheat the Instant Pot to the sauté function. When it's hot, add the canola oil. Season the pork shoulder with salt and pepper. Sear on all sides until well browned, about 10 minutes total. Add the onion, garlic, and salsa verde. Cover and pressure cook for 35 minutes.
2. Shred the pork with a fork and adjust seasoning. Divide between serving bowls.
3. Top with mozzarella, avocado, sour cream, green onions, and cilantro.

COOKING TIP: Make sure to switch to pressure cooking, not sautéing when you place the lid on the Instant Pot.

NUTRITION PER SERVING

CALORIES: 612 FAT: 46g PROTEIN: 35g TOTAL CARBS: 12g FIBER: 3g NET CARBS: 9g

Roasted Pork Tenderloin with Cabbage Slaw over Mashed Cauliflower GF NF

Vibrant purple cabbage retains its crispness over creamy mashed cauliflower with oven-roasted pork tenderloin in this comfort food bowl. Serve with a glass of crisp white wine or pinot noir.

YIELD: 4 servings | **PREP TIME:** 10 minutes | **COOK TIME:** 20 minutes

2 tablespoons canola oil, divided

1½ pounds pork tenderloin

sea salt

freshly ground pepper

1 tablespoon minced rosemary

1 small head cabbage, thinly sliced

1 small red onion, thinly sliced

1 tablespoon apple cider vinegar

½ cup roughly chopped flat-leaf parsley

1 recipe Mashed Cauliflower (page 98)

1. Preheat the oven to 425°F.
2. Heat a large ovenproof skillet over medium-high heat. Add 1 tablespoon of the oil and tilt to coat the pan.
3. Dry the pork tenderloin with paper towels and season with salt and pepper and the rosemary. Sear the pork until browned on all sides, about 10 minutes total.
4. Transfer to the oven and roast for another 10 minutes, or until the pork is cooked through.
5. Transfer the pork to a cutting board to rest.
6. Add the cabbage and onion to the pan and toss gently, allowing the residual heat of the pan to wilt the cabbage. Add the apple cider vinegar and parsley to the pan and toss gently to mix.
7. Divide the mashed cauliflower between serving bowls. Top with the cabbage slaw.
8. Slice the pork on a bias and divide between serving bowls.

NUTRITION PER SERVING

CALORIES: 574 TOTAL FAT: 30g PROTEIN: 53g CARBOHYDRATES: 19g FIBER: 8g NET CARBS: 11g

Pork Panzanella GF NF

If you're familiar with traditional panzanella, I'm sorry for my appropriation of the word. The traditional Italian salad uses stale bread cubes to soak up the juices from fresh tomatoes, herbs, oil, and vinegar. In this keto version, pork takes the place of bread, making it a full meal with many of the flavors of the original. It's perfect in late summer and an ideal way to use up leftover pork roast, tenderloin, or pork chops.

YIELD: 2 servings | **PREP TIME:** 10 minutes | **COOK TIME:** 0 minutes

- 8 ounces cooked pork tenderloin, cut into bite-size pieces
- 4 ounces fresh mozzarella, cut into bite-size pieces
- 2 plum tomatoes, diced
- ½ cup diced cucumber
- ¼ cup minced fresh basil
- 2 tablespoons extra-virgin olive oil
- 2 teaspoons balsamic vinegar
- sea salt
- freshly ground pepper

1. Combine the pork, mozzarella, tomatoes, cucumber, basil, olive oil, and vinegar in a mixing bowl. Season with salt and pepper.
2. Divide between serving bowls. Serve chilled.

NUTRITION PER SERVING

CALORIES: 534 TOTAL FAT: 36g PROTEIN: 47g CARBOHYDRATES: 5g FIBER: 1g NET CARBS: 4g

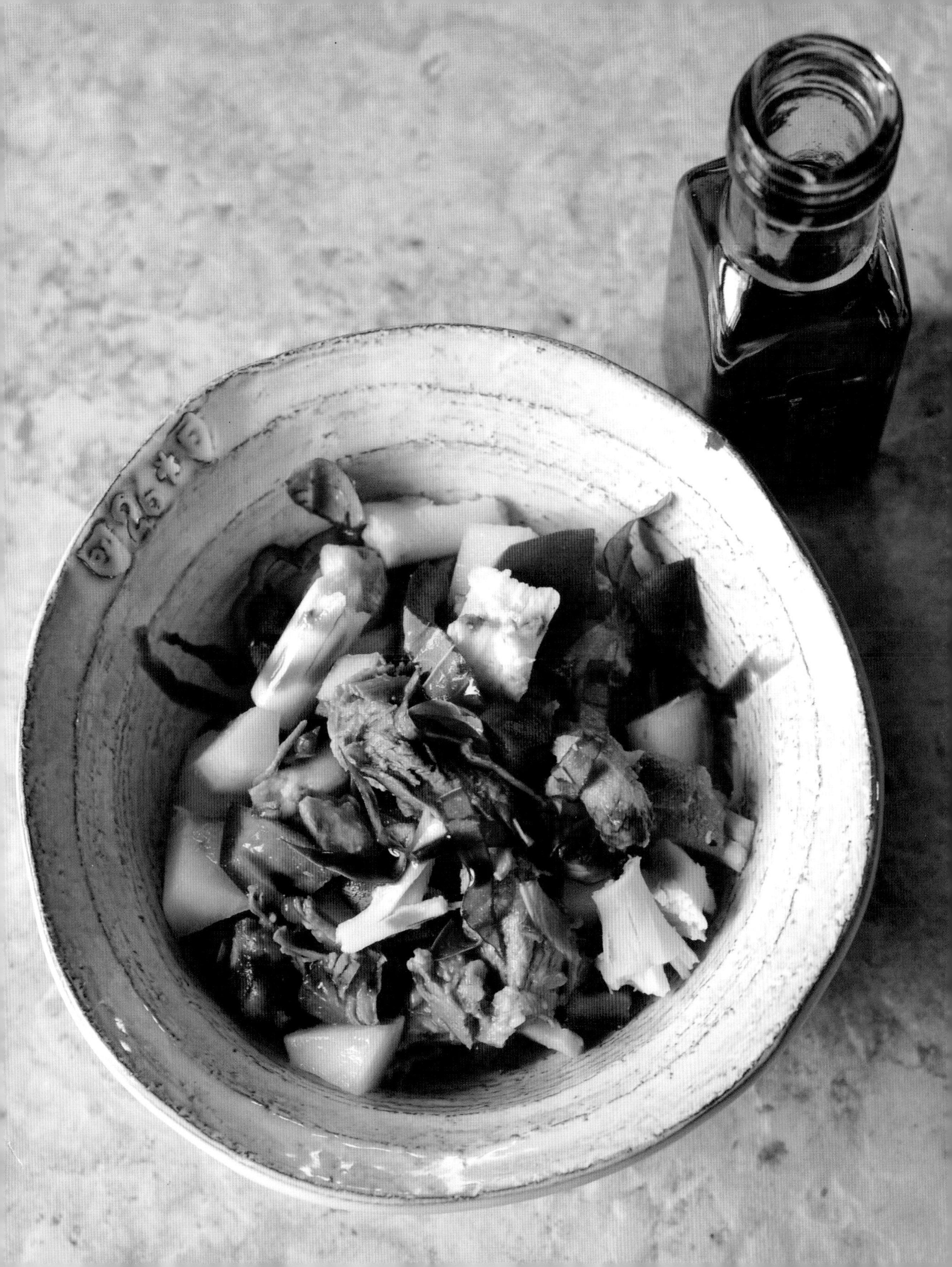

CHAPTER SEVEN

VEGETARIAN

My husband, Rich, has been a vegetarian since I've known him. So when I cook for the two of us, it's always sans meat. That has certainly challenged my culinary skills—I expect my meatless meals to taste as good or maybe even better than meaty main dishes. This chapter has some of my favorites, including a way to prepare tofu that will have you totally rethinking the plant-based protein.

- Curried Cauliflower and Tofu Bowls with Arugula
- Ratatouille and Goat Cheese Bowls
- Vibrant Tofu Carrot Noodle Bowls
- Keto Bibimbap
- Tempeh Taco Bowls with Avocado, Cherry Tomato, and Lime Vinaigrette
- Egg Roll Scramble

Curried Cauliflower and Tofu Bowls with Arugula GF V

Curry-spiced roasted cauliflower, arugula, and tofu make a large and filling meal for just a few calories. The tahini yogurt dressing is addicting and it's worth making a double batch to have more on hand for other salads or for dipping vegetables. To make it vegan, use a plant-based yogurt.

YIELD: 4 servings | **PREP TIME:** 10 minutes | **COOK TIME:** 20 to 25 minutes

- 1 small head cauliflower, broken into florets
- 1 tablespoon curry powder
- 2 tablespoons canola oil, divided
- 1 block tofu, drained and pressed, cut into 1-inch cubes
- sea salt
- freshly ground pepper
- 1 cup whole-milk, plain yogurt
- ¼ cup tahini
- 1 teaspoon minced fresh garlic
- 1 tablespoon extra-virgin olive oil
- 2 tablespoons lemon juice
- 2 cups arugula
- ½ cup sliced almonds

1. Preheat the oven to 400°F. Place the cauliflower florets into a bowl and season with the curry powder and 1 tablespoon of the canola oil. Spread the cauliflower onto half of a baking sheet lined with parchment paper.
2. Place the tofu into the same bowl used for the cauliflower and drizzle with the remaining tablespoon of oil. Season with salt and pepper. Spread the tofu onto the remaining half of the baking sheet. Bake for 15 minutes. Flip the cauliflower and tofu and bake for another 5 to 10 minutes, or until the tofu is gently browned and the cauliflower is soft.
3. While the cauliflower and tofu cook, whisk the yogurt, tahini, garlic, olive oil, and lemon juice in a small jar. Season with salt.
4. Divide the cauliflower and tofu between serving bowls. Add the arugula and drizzle the yogurt tahini dressing over it. Top with the sliced almonds.

COOKING TIP: To press tofu, slice the block in half horizontally. Place the slabs on a cutting board with space between them. Top with a second cutting board and then place something heavy, such as a cast-iron skillet, on top. Set the cutting boards near the kitchen sink and allow the water to seep out for about 15 minutes.

NUTRITION PER SERVING

CALORIES: 377 TOTAL FAT: 31g PROTEIN: 17g CARBOHYDRATES: 15g FIBER: 6g NET CARBS: 9g

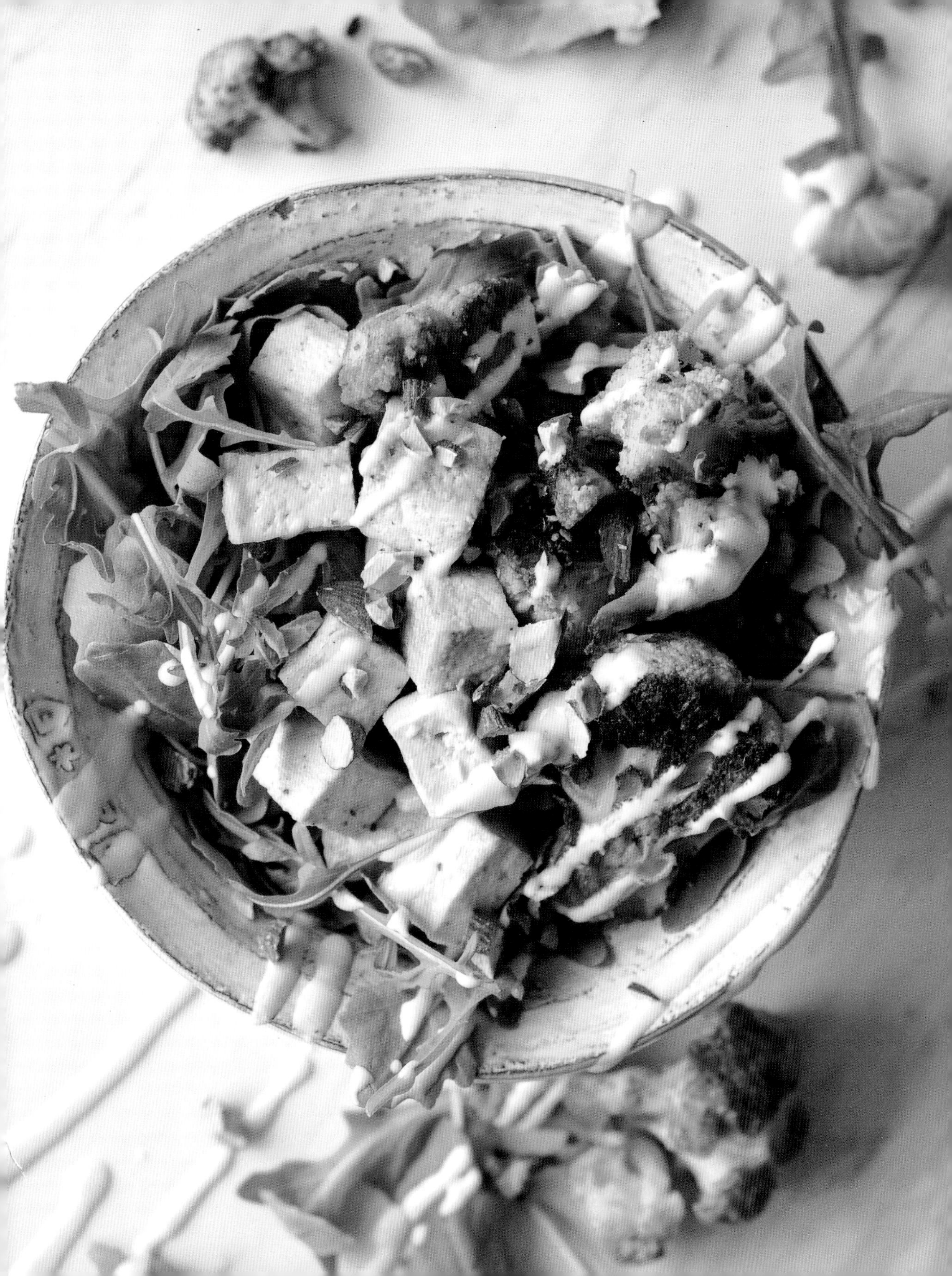

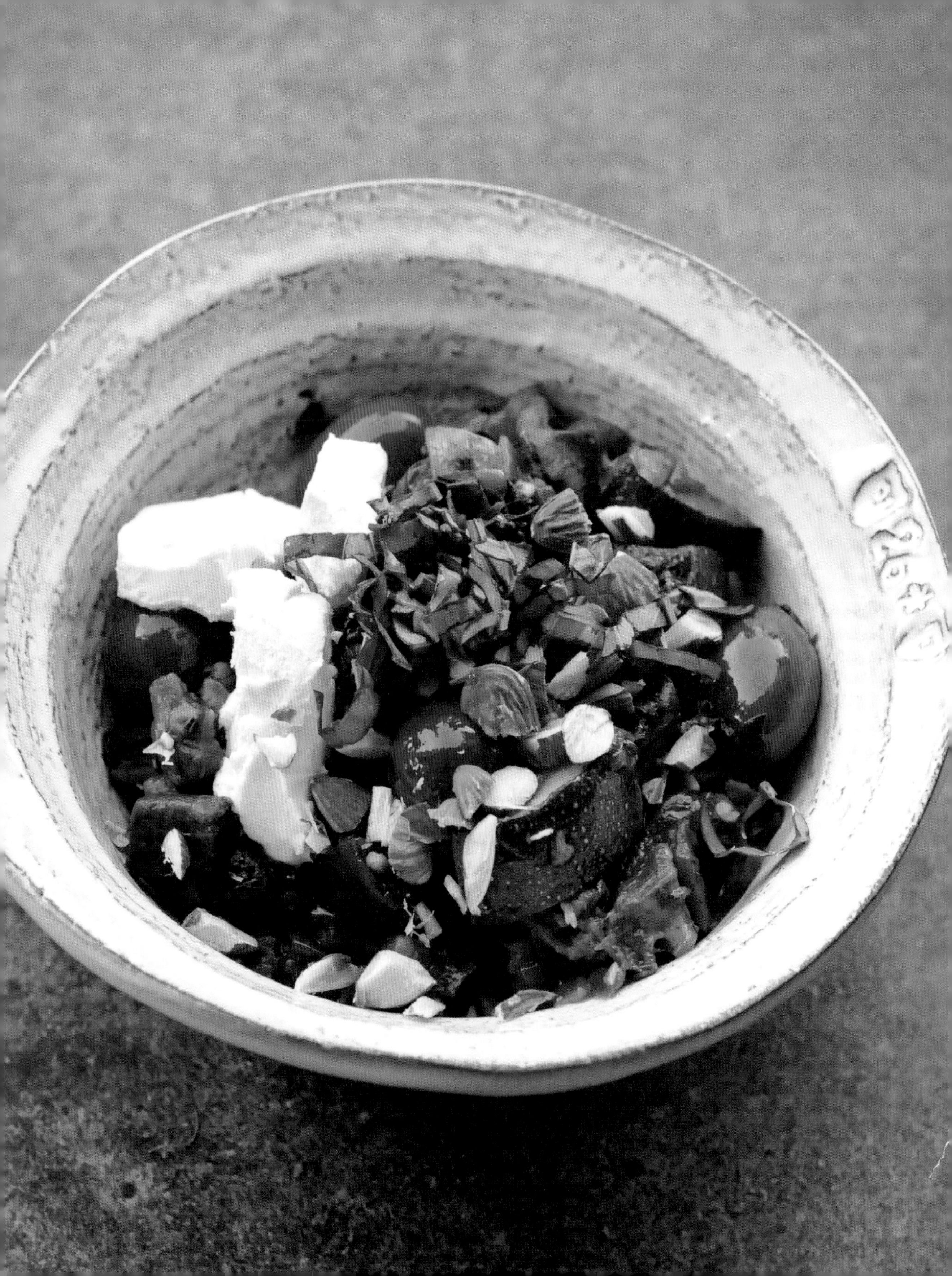

Ratatouille and Goat Cheese Bowls GF V

Succulent roasted eggplant, zucchini, and tomatoes are roasted in olive oil and herbs in this comfort food bowl. The recipe calls for goat cheese. Vegan nut-based cheeses are also delicious here. The cooking time might seem long, but it's all hands off. The flavors of this dish improve with time, so it's also awesome for meal prepping; just keep the cheese separate until ready to serve.

YIELD: 4 servings | **PREP TIME:** 10 minutes | **COOK TIME:** 40 to 45 minutes

- 1 small eggplant, sliced in ¼-inch rounds
- 2 plum tomatoes, sliced in ¼-inch rounds
- 2 medium zucchini, sliced in ¼-inch rounds
- ¼ cup extra-virgin olive oil
- 1 teaspoon fresh thyme leaves
- ½ cup roughly chopped fresh basil, plus more for garnish
- sea salt
- freshly ground pepper
- 8 ounces goat cheese
- ¼ cup toasted pine nuts

1. Preheat the oven to 375°F. Place the eggplant, tomatoes, zucchini, oil, thyme, and basil in a large bowl. Season with salt and pepper. Toss gently to coat the vegetables in the oil.
2. Arrange the vegetables in a casserole dish, cover tightly with a lid or foil, and bake for 30 minutes. Remove the foil and bake for another 10 to 15 minutes, or until the vegetables are tender and beginning to brown.
3. Divide the vegetables between serving bowls. Top with crumbled goat cheese and pine nuts.

NUTRITION PER SERVING

CALORIES: 363 TOTAL FAT: 30g PROTEIN: 13g CARBOHYDRATES: 13g FIBER: 5g NET CARBS: 8g

Vibrant Tofu Carrot Noodle Bowls NF Vg

YIELD: 4 servings | **PREP TIME:** 15 minutes | **COOK TIME:** 20 minutes

1 (14-ounce) block extra-firm tofu (not silken), sliced in half horizontally

2 tablespoons toasted sesame oil, divided

¼ cup low-sodium soy sauce

2 tablespoons lime juice

2 tablespoons neutral oil, such as avocado or canola oil

1 to 3 teaspoons sambal oelek chili paste or 1 teaspoon minced red chili

1 to 3 drops liquid stevia

¼ head green cabbage, shredded

2 large carrots, peeled, spiralized or sliced thinly with a vegetable peeler

large handful roughly chopped fresh mint

large handful roughly chopped fresh basil

large handful roughly chopped cilantro

4 tablespoons toasted sesame seeds

1. Preheat the oven to 425°F.
2. Place the two slabs of tofu between two cutting boards and top with a cast-iron skillet or something else heavy. Allow the water to seep from the tofu for at least 5 minutes. Cut the tofu into about 1-inch cubes.
3. Place the tofu cubes into a bowl and toss with 1 tablespoon of sesame oil. Spread the tofu onto a rimmed baking sheet and bake for 15 minutes. Flip the tofu and cook for another 5 minutes.
4. To make the dressing, combine the remaining sesame oil, soy sauce, lime juice, avocado or other oil, chili paste, and stevia in a small jar. Cover with a lid and shake to combine.
5. To assemble, divide the cabbage, carrot noodles, herbs, and roasted tofu between four serving bowls and drizzle with the dressing. Toss gently to mix and top with the sesame seeds.

NUTRITION PER SERVING

CALORIES: 310 TOTAL FAT: 25g PROTEIN: 15g CARBOHYDRATES: 12g FIBER: 5g NET CARBS: 7g

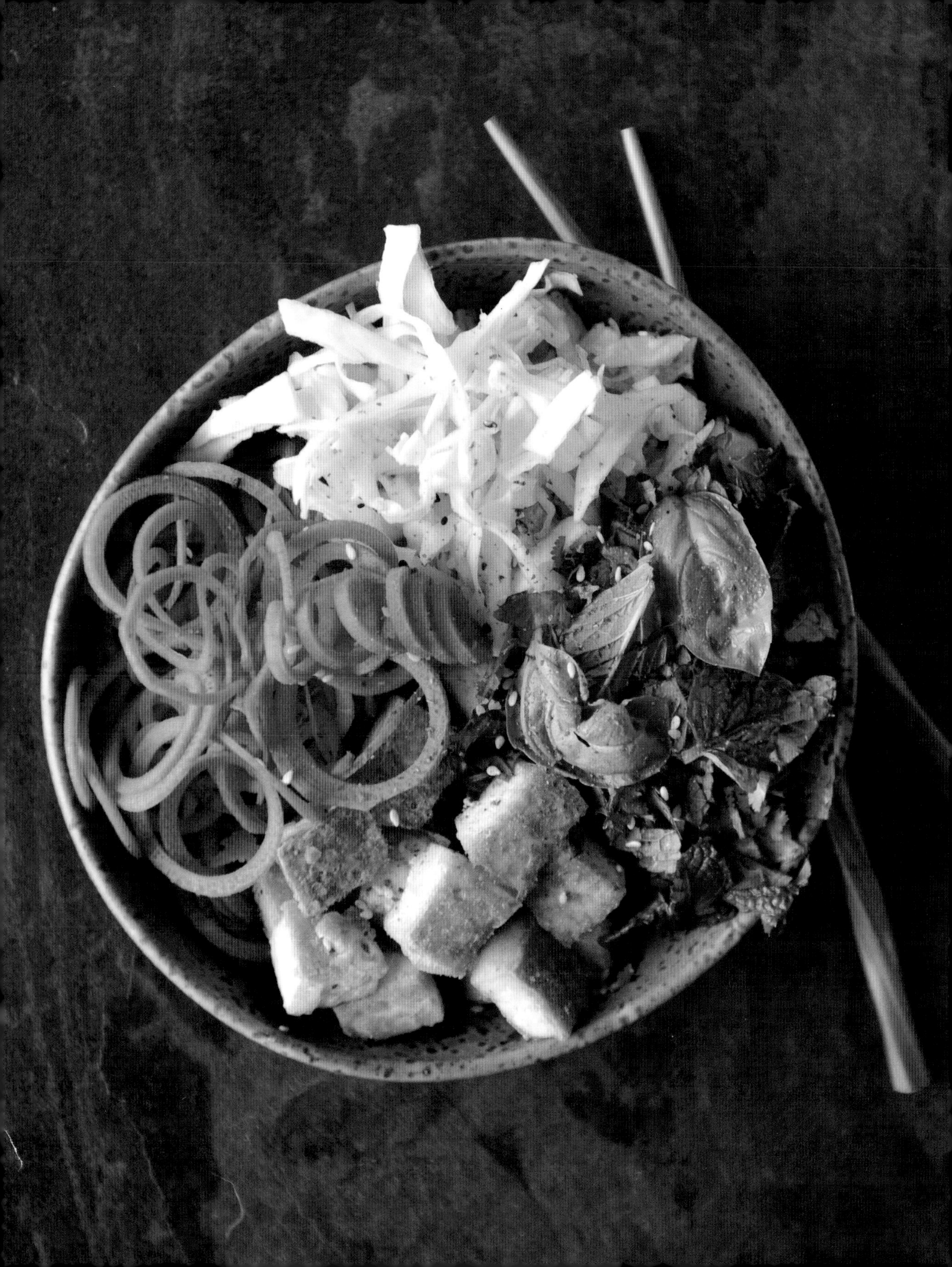

Keto Bibimbap DF GF NF V

Korean rice bowls might not sound like a low-carb meal, but once you replace the rice with cauliflower, you'll see how keto-friendly it is. Most bibimbap is served with kimchi, and if that's your thing, go for it! If not, make this simple quick-pickled cabbage as a tangy topping. It's not the same thing, but it does the job.

YIELD: 2 servings | **PREP TIME:** 10 minutes | **COOK TIME:** 6 to 8 minutes

- 1 tablespoon chili garlic sauce
- ¼ cup rice vinegar
- ½ teaspoon sea salt
- 2 cups shredded green cabbage
- 1 tablespoon canola oil
- 4 eggs
- 1 recipe Cauli Rice (page 100)
- 1 tablespoon toasted sesame oil, plus more for drizzling
- 4 cups fresh spinach
- ½ teaspoon minced garlic
- 2 green onions, white and green parts, thinly sliced
- ¼ cup shredded carrot

1. To make the quick-pickled cauliflower, whisk the chili garlic sauce, vinegar, and sea salt in a small bowl. Add the cabbage and toss gently to coat. Set aside.
2. Heat the canola oil in a large skillet over medium-high heat. Pan fry the eggs for 5 to 7 minutes, or until the whites are set and the yolks reach your desired consistency.
3. Divide the Cauli Rice between serving bowls. Top each with two fried eggs.
4. Return the skillet to the heat. Add the sesame oil, spinach, and garlic. Cook for about 1 minute, or just until the spinach is wilted. Transfer it to the serving bowls.
5. Top with the green onions, a spoonful of the quick-pickled cabbage, and a few carrot pieces.

NUTRITION PER SERVING

CALORIES: 367 TOTAL FAT: 28g PROTEIN: 19g CARBOHYDRATES: 15g FIBER: 8g NET CARBS: 7g

Tempeh Taco Bowls with Avocado, Cherry Tomato, and Lime Vinaigrette DF GF NF Vg

Tempeh stands in for ground beef in this yummy deconstructed taco bowl. Instead of guacamole and pico de gallo, this one features a cherry tomato and avocado salad with lime dressing. Serve the whole thing over a bed of lettuce.

YIELD: 4 servings | **PREP TIME:** 10 minutes | **COOK TIME:** 4 minutes

- 1 tablespoon canola oil
- 8 ounces tempeh
- 1 tablespoon taco seasoning or chili powder
- sea salt
- freshly ground pepper
- 1 tablespoon extra-virgin olive oil
- 2 tablespoons lime juice
- 2 large avocados, diced
- 1 pint cherry tomatoes, halved
- 4 cups shredded romaine lettuce

1. Heat the oil in a medium skillet over medium-high heat. Break the tempeh into pieces and stir-fry for 3 minutes, until beginning to brown. Add the taco seasoning, salt, and pepper. Cook for another minute. Set aside.
2. Whisk the olive oil and lime juice together in a bowl. Season with salt. Add the avocados and tomatoes and toss gently to coat them in the dressing.
3. Divide the lettuce between serving bowls. Top with the avocado-tomato salad and the tempeh taco meat.

COOKING TIP: The carbs might seem high, but nearly half of them are from the fiber in the avocados.

NUTRITION PER SERVING

CALORIES: 341 TOTAL FAT: 27g PROTEIN: 14g CARBOHYDRATES: 17g FIBER: 8g NET CARBS: 9g

Egg Roll Scramble DF NF V

I took a few liberties with the classic egg rolls. This one is low carb, vegetarian, and in a bowl (obviously), and I scrambled eggs into the mix. That said, it has all the flavors you love in classic egg rolls.

YIELD: 2 servings | **PREP TIME:** 10 minutes | **COOK TIME:** 10 minutes

2 tablespoons canola oil

1 small red onion, halved and thinly sliced

1 small carrot, peeled, julienned

2 cups roughly chopped mushrooms

1 teaspoon minced fresh garlic

2 tablespoons soy sauce

4 cups shredded cabbage

1 tablespoon toasted sesame oil

4 eggs, whisked

2 teaspoons rice wine vinegar

2 green onions, green parts, thinly sliced

1. Heat the canola oil in a large skillet. Add the onion and carrot and sauté for 2 minutes. Add the mushrooms and cook for another 3 minutes. Add the garlic, soy sauce, and cabbage and sauté for another 2 minutes.
2. Push the vegetables to the sides of the pan and add the sesame oil, then the eggs. Stir-fry until just cooked, about 3 minutes, then fold everything together and season with the vinegar. Divide between serving bowls and top with the green onions.

NUTRITION PER SERVING

CALORIES: 380 TOTAL FAT: 32g PROTEIN: 16g CARBOHYDRATES: 11g FIBER: 4g NET CARBS: 7g

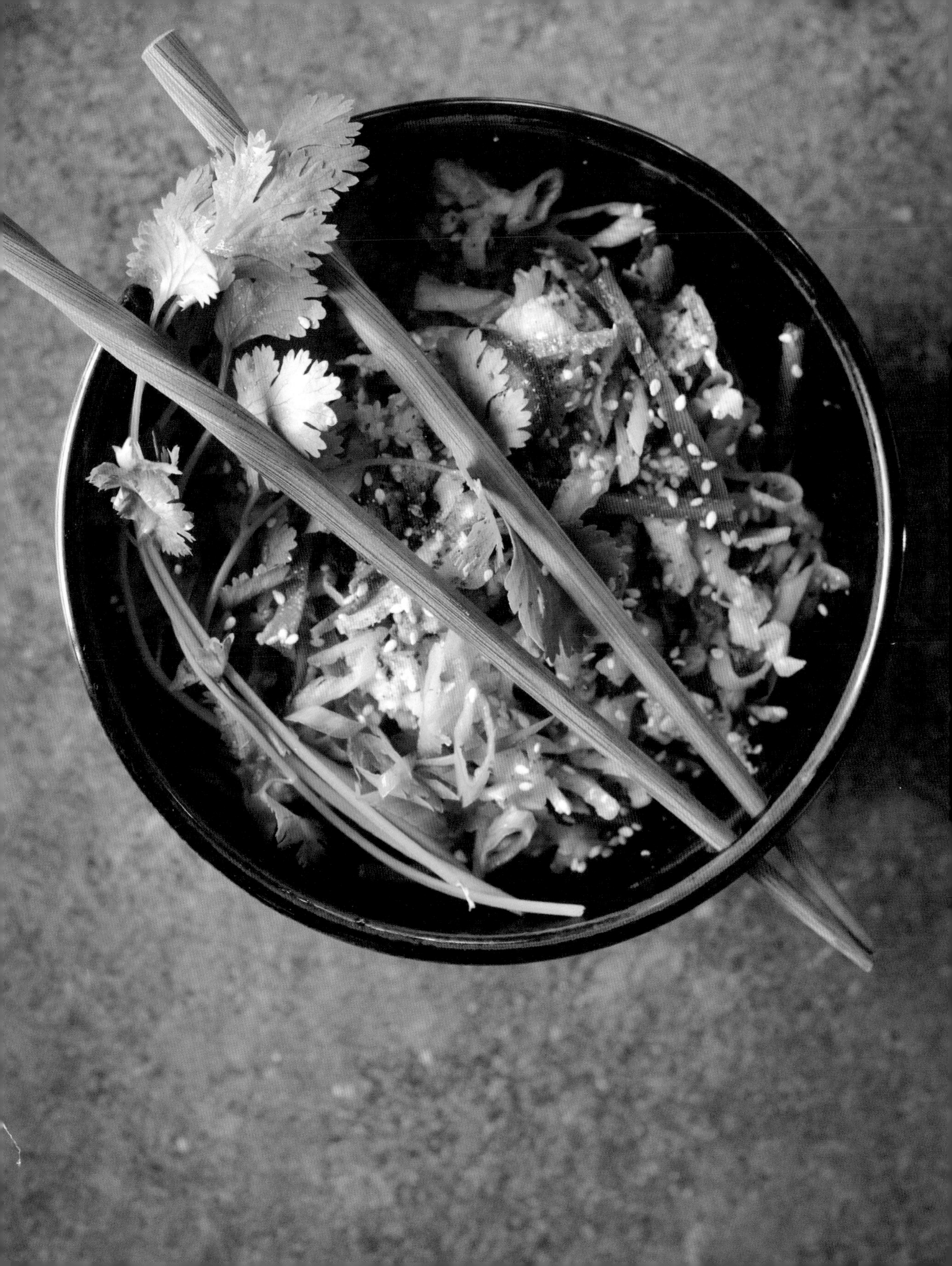

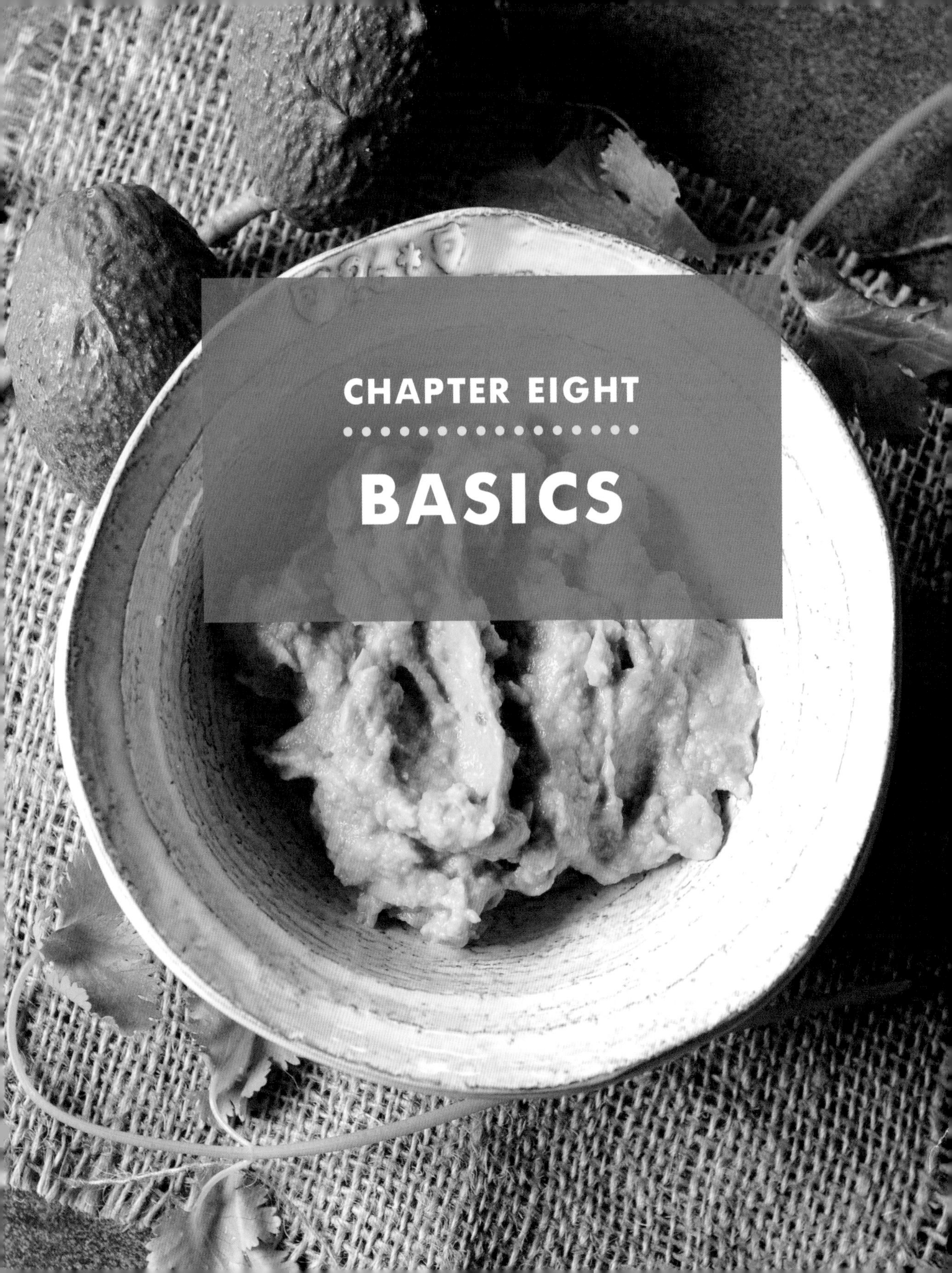

CHAPTER EIGHT

BASICS

If you're new to keto, even the most basic tasks are new to you. Making noodles with vegetables and roasting spaghetti squash aren't exactly mainstream cookbook fare. Fortunately, once you get the hang of it, you'll wonder why it took you so long to give these easy-peasy, low-carb staples a try.

- Mashed Cauliflower
- Cauli Rice
- Spaghetti Squash
- Vegetable Noodles
- Guacamole
- Pico de Gallo
- Salsa Verde
- Celeriac Puree
- Lemon Herb Vinaigrette
- Balsamic Vinaigrette

Mashed Cauliflower GF NF V

I'll be honest with you—before I tried mashed cauliflower, I thought there was absolutely no way it could hold a candle to real mashed potatoes. Boy, was I mistaken! With a little salt and butter, it's just like the real thing, but it doesn't leave you with a carb hangover. This mashed cauli recipe forms the basis for many of the comfort food bowls in this book.

YIELD: 4 servings | **PREP TIME:** 5 minutes | **COOK TIME:** 10 minutes

- 1 head cauliflower, cored and cut into florets
- ¼ cup whole milk
- 3 tablespoons butter
- ½ teaspoon garlic powder
- 1 teaspoon sea salt

1. Place the cauliflower in a large pot with about ½ inch of water. Cover and steam for 10 minutes, or until the cauliflower is very tender. Drain, reserving the cooking liquid.
2. Transfer the cauliflower to a blender along with the milk, butter, garlic powder, and sea salt. Puree until smooth, scraping down the sides as needed. Add additional cooking liquid as needed to reach your desired consistency. Store in a covered container in the refrigerator for up to 2 days.

COOKING TIP: For a dairy-free version, use unsweetened, plain almond milk and Earth Balance Buttery Spread or another vegan butter.

NUTRITION PER SERVING

CALORIES: 122 TOTAL FAT: 9g PROTEIN: 3g CARBOHYDRATES: 8g FIBER: 4g NET CARBS: 4g

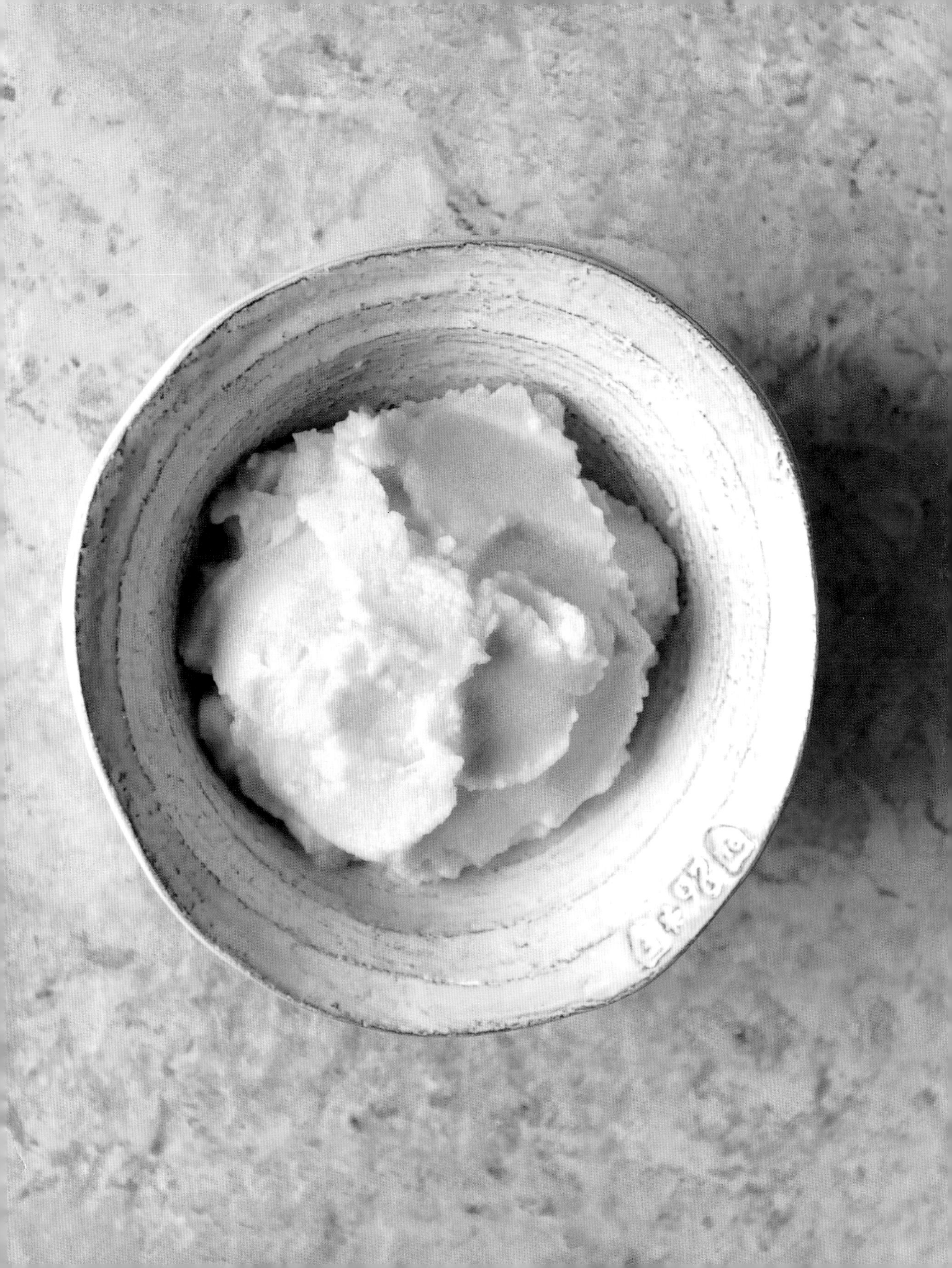

Cauli Rice DF GF NF Vg

Cauli rice serves as a tasty and filling low-carb stand-in for traditional white rice. It has 75 percent fewer calories than rice and only 3 grams of net carbs per serving.

YIELD: 4 servings | **PREP TIME:** 5 minutes | **COOK TIME:** 5 minutes

1 medium head cauliflower, cored and cut into florets

1 tablespoon coconut oil or canola oil

sea salt

1. Process the cauliflower in a food processor until it resembles small grains of rice. Cook immediately, or store in a covered container in the refrigerator for up to 3 days.
2. Heat a large skillet over medium-high heat. Add the coconut oil.
3. Sauté the cauliflower until it is al dente, about 5 minutes. Season with salt.

NUTRITION PER SERVING

CALORIES: 67 TOTAL FAT: 4g PROTEIN: 3g CARBOHYDRATES: 7g FIBER: 4g NET CARBS: 3g

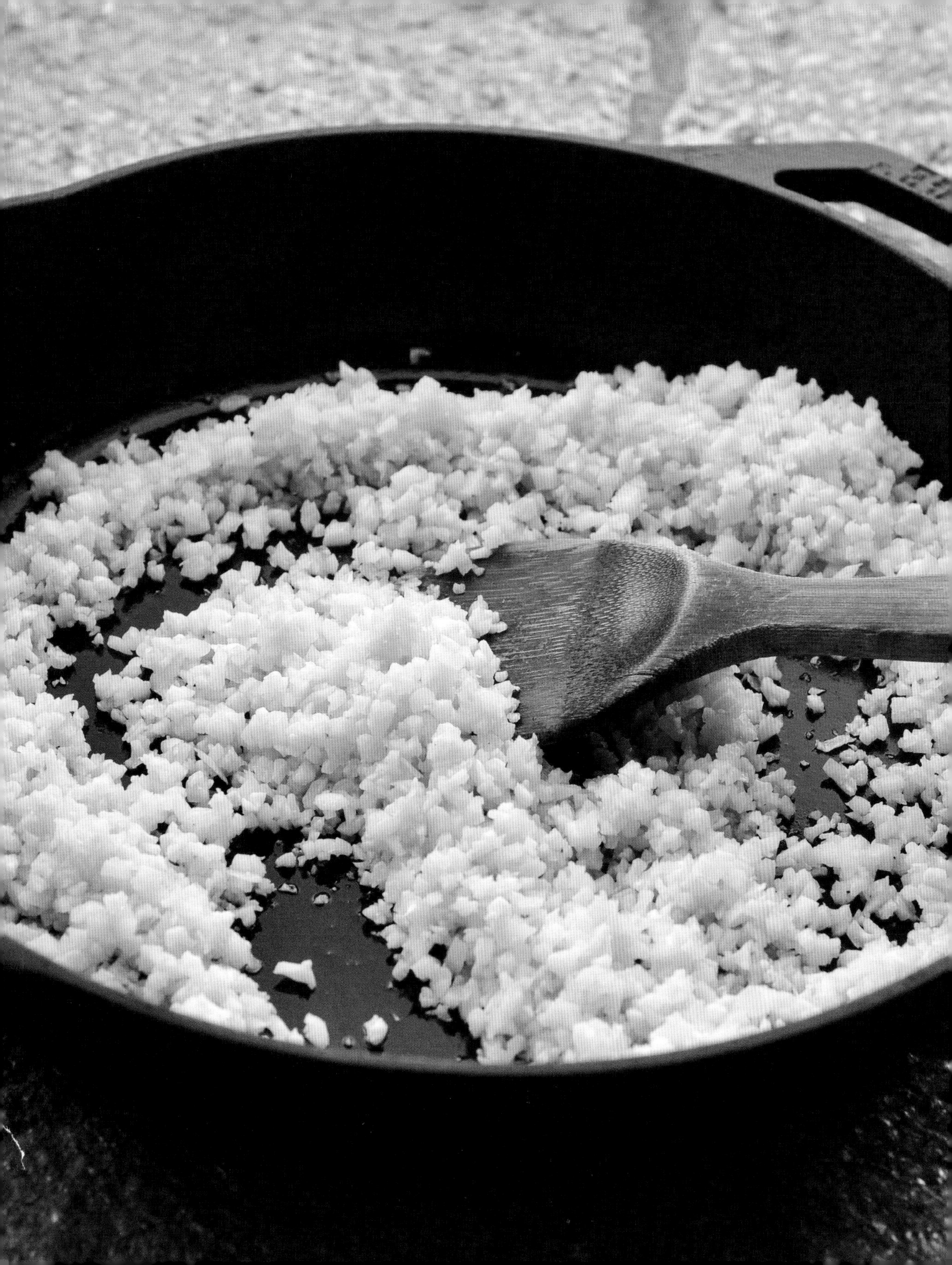

Spaghetti Squash DF GF NF Vg

Like its name suggests, spaghetti squash is the perfect low-carb stand-in for spaghetti. The trick to getting the longest strands is to slice the squash into rounds. Use it wherever you might use pasta noodles.

YIELD: 4 servings | **PREP TIME:** 5 minutes | **COOK TIME:** 20 to 25 minutes

1 spaghetti squash, sliced into 1-inch-thick rounds, seeds and strings cut

1. Preheat the oven to 375°F.
2. Spread the squash onto a rimmed baking sheet.
3. Roast for 20 to 25 minutes, or until the squash is tender. Use a fork to scrape the squash away from the skin. Try to do this in one stroke, around the center of the squash to get the longest noodles. Store in a covered container in the refrigerator for up to 2 days.

NUTRITION PER SERVING

CALORIES: 36 TOTAL FAT: 0g PROTEIN: 1g CARBOHYDRATES: 8g FIBER: 2g NET CARBS: 6g

Vegetable Noodles DF GF NF Vg

Zucchini, carrots, cucumber, even jicama works to make vegetable noodles. Really, the only consideration is to make sure whatever veggie you use is 1½–2 inches thick and isn't hollow. Some vegetables do best if you sweat them first, which means to salt generously, allow to rest in a colander, then rinse and squeeze out excess moisture. For zucchini, this helps the vegetable stay firm and chewy when cooked. Other vegetables are best served raw. Use your judgment and consider the flavor and texture you want in your finished dish.

YIELD: 4 servings | **PREP TIME:** 5 minutes | **COOK TIME:** 2 to 3 minutes

1 pound vegetables suitable for spiralizing

sea salt

olive oil

1. If the vegetable is long, such as a carrot or zucchini, slice in half and slice off the stem ends.
2. Place one end of the vegetable onto the spiky side of the handle-end of your spiralizer. Slide the device so the opposite end is near the blade. Turn the handle to slice the vegetable into noodles. Repeat with the remaining vegetables. Cook immediately, or store in a covered container in the refrigerator for up to 3 days.
3. For cooked noodles: Generously salt the noodles and place them into a colander to rest for 10 to 15 minutes. Rinse under cold water and squeeze to remove excess moisture.
4. Heat a sauté pan over medium-high heat. Add 1 tablespoon of oil. Sauté the noodles for 2 to 3 minutes, or until cooked to your desired consistency. This will vary depending on the vegetable you choose.

NUTRITION PER SERVING (FOR ZUCCHINI NOODLES COOKED WITH OIL)

CALORIES: 48 TOTAL FAT: 3g PROTEIN: 1g CARBOHYDRATES: 4g FIBER: 2g NET CARBS: 2g

Guacamole DF GF NF Vg

Avocado is one of my favorite fruits, and it grows abundantly in Santa Barbara, where I live. I like to purchase it from a lovely woman who lives down the street from me. It's naturally low in carbs (it has some, but mostly fiber) and high in fat—making it the perfect plant-based addition to your keto bowl meal.

YIELD: 2 cups (serving size 2 tablespoons) | **PREP TIME:** 5 minutes | **COOK TIME:** 0 minutes

4 large ripe avocados, diced

½ teaspoon minced fresh garlic

2 tablespoons lime juice

sea salt

2 tablespoons minced cilantro

Place the avocado, garlic, and lime juice into a mortar and pestle and mash until it reaches your desired consistency. Season to taste with salt. Stir in the cilantro, if using. Store in a bowl tightly covered with plastic wrap (the wrap should be pressed against the guacamole) in the refrigerator for up to 1 day.

NUTRITION PER SERVING

CALORIES: 70 TOTAL FAT: 7g PROTEIN: 1g CARBOHYDRATES: 3g FIBER: 2g NET CARBS: 1g

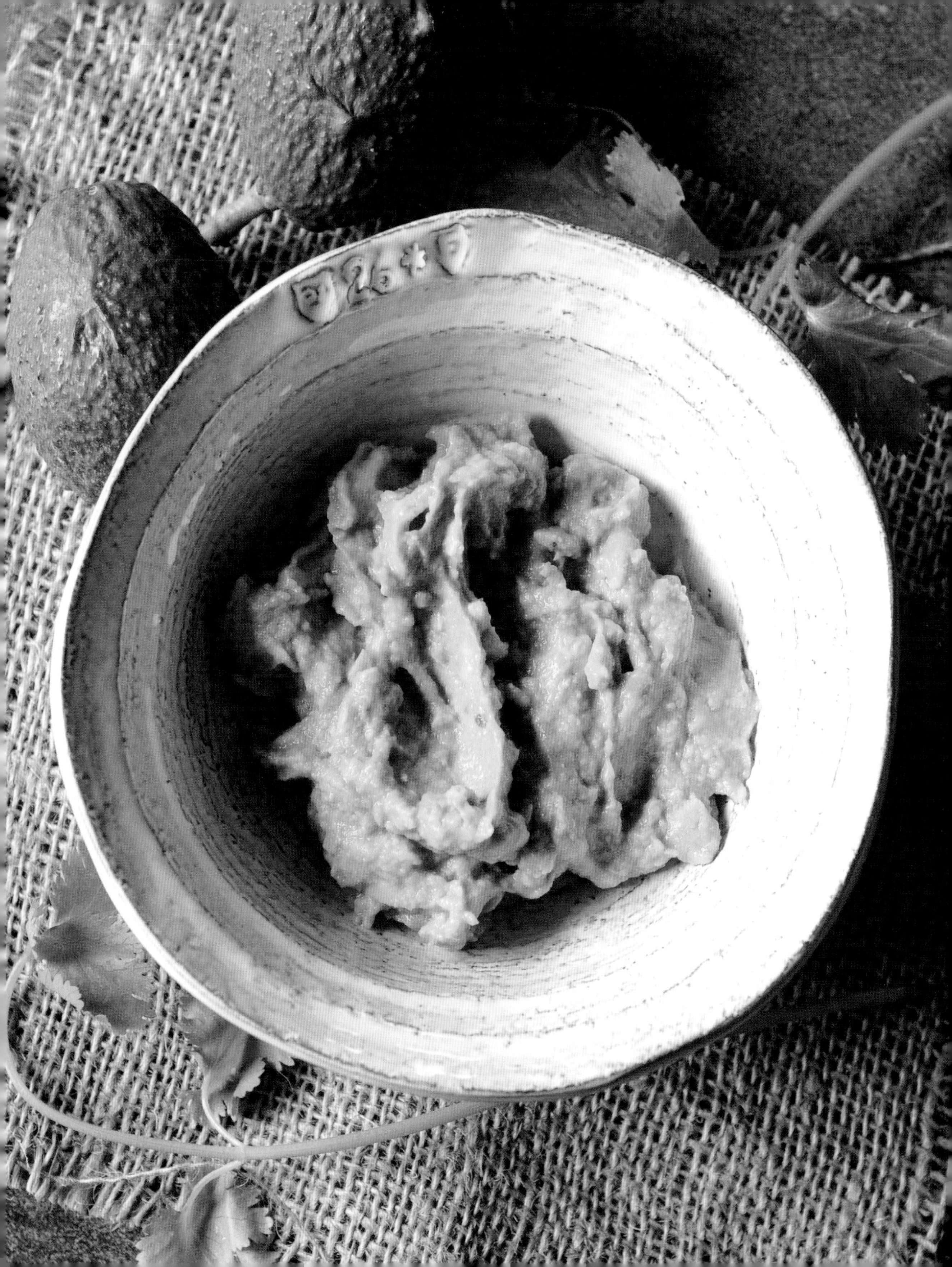

Pico de Gallo DF GF NF Vg

When I was a child, my parents bought a "salsa maker" from an infomercial. This put salsa into the realm of complicated and expensive. First, you had to blanch the tomatoes, and then use the special chopping device that would cut them without blitzing them into a sauce. What a hassle! First, there's no need to remove the tomato skins. Second, you know what else chops and dices? A good chef's knife! Save your money and use it to buy the freshest heirloom tomatoes you can at your local farmers market.

YIELD: 6 (½-cup) servings | **PREP TIME:** 5 minutes

- 2 cups diced tomatoes
- ½ cup diced red onion
- ½ cup minced cilantro
- 1 tablespoon minced jalapeno
- 2 tablespoons lime juice
- sea salt
- freshly ground pepper

In a large bowl, mix the tomatoes, onion, cilantro, jalapeno, and lime juice. Season with salt and pepper. Store in a covered container in the refrigerator for up to 2 days.

NUTRITION PER SERVING

CALORIES: 20 TOTAL FAT: 0g PROTEIN: 0g CARBOHYDRATES: 4g FIBER: 2g NET CARBS: 2g

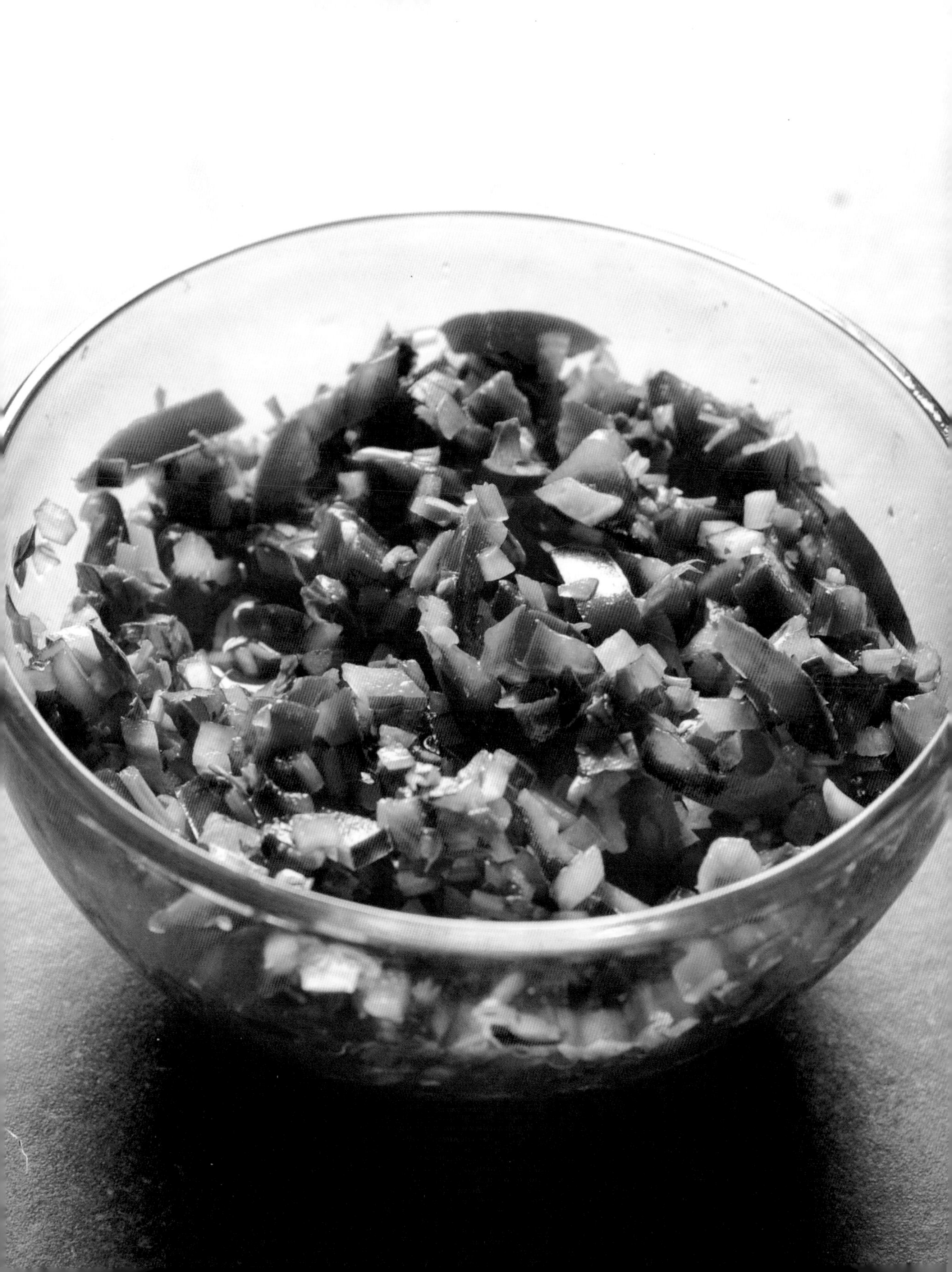

Salsa Verde DF GF NF Vg

I can't think of a better word than "punchy" for this salsa. The spicy jalapeno, herbal cilantro, and tangy lime juice marry for a creamy sauce that livens up whatever you pour it on. It goes really well with chorizo and Cauli Rice (page 100).

YIELD: 4 (2-tablespoon) servings | **PREP TIME:** 5 minutes | **COOK TIME:** 0 minutes

- 1 large jalapeno pepper, seeded and minced
- 1 cup packed minced cilantro
- 2 tablespoons fresh lime juice, from 1 to 2 limes
- ½ teaspoon sea salt
- 2 tablespoons extra-virgin olive oil

Place all of the ingredients into a blender and puree until mostly smooth. Store in a covered container in the refrigerator for up to 2 days.

NUTRITION PER SERVING

CALORIES: 36 TOTAL FAT: 4g PROTEIN: 1g CARBOHYDRATES: 1g FIBER: 1g NET CARBS: 0g

Celeriac Puree GF NF V

As much as I love cauliflower, sometimes it's nice to get a change of pace from the cruciferous vegetable. Enter celeriac. It's a root vegetable, but it has a fraction of the carbs of potatoes.

YIELD: 4 servings | **PREP TIME:** 5 minutes | **COOK TIME:** 20 minutes

- 1 large celery root, peeled and diced
- ½ cup milk
- ½ teaspoon sea salt
- ¼ cup butter

Place the celery root, milk, and sea salt into a pot set over medium-low heat. Cover with a lid and simmer for 20 minutes. Drain the celery root and transfer to a food processor along with the butter. Puree until smooth. Store in a covered container in the refrigerator for up to 2 days.

COOKING TIP: Don't even think about trying to use a vegetable peeler with celeriac. Instead, brush away the dirt as much as you can, and use a sharp chef's knife to slice away the tough peel. You should get roughly 4 cups of diced celery root for this recipe.

NUTRITION PER SERVING

CALORIES: 162 TOTAL FAT: 13g PROTEIN: 3g CARBOHYDRATES: 10g FIBER: 2g NET CARBS: 8g

Lemon Herb Vinaigrette DF GF NF Vg

This is my go-to blended salad dressing. It's creamy, savory, herbal, and subtly tangy. Serve it with … everything!

YIELD: 8 (2-tablespoon) servings | **PREP TIME:** 5 minutes | **COOK TIME:** 0 minutes

1 cup roughly chopped fresh parsley

2 tablespoons minced assorted fresh herbs, such as basil, thyme, and tarragon

½ bunch green onions, trimmed, roughly chopped, or 2 peeled shallots, roughly chopped

2 garlic cloves, roughly chopped

1 teaspoon Dijon mustard

1 to 2 drops liquid stevia, to taste

zest and juice of 2 lemons

1 tablespoon white wine vinegar

½ cup extra-virgin olive oil

½ teaspoon kosher salt

Place all of the ingredients into a blender and puree until smooth. Store in a covered container in the refrigerator for up to 2 days.

NUTRITION PER SERVING

CALORIES: 124 TOTAL FAT: 14g PROTEIN: 0g CARBOHYDRATES: 1g FIBER: 1g NET CARBS: 0g

Balsamic Vinaigrette DF GF NF

My brother lived in Italy for several years and sent me a selection of good balsamic vinegars one year for my birthday. Vinegar might sound like an odd gift, but I was thrilled. Try to get your hands on the best balsamic and extra-virgin olive oil that you can for this recipe—it really does make a difference!

YIELD: 8 (2-tablespoon) servings | **PREP TIME:** 10 minutes | **COOK TIME:** 30 minutes

⅓ cup balsamic vinegar
1 teaspoon honey
¼ teaspoon Dijon mustard
1 shallot, minced
1 tablespoon minced basil
sea salt
freshly ground pepper
⅔ cup extra-virgin olive oil

1. Place the vinegar, honey, mustard, shallot, and basil in a bowl. Season generously with salt and pepper.
2. Whisk in the olive oil slowly until it comes together in a thick emulsion. Season to taste with additional salt and pepper.

NUTRITION PER SERVING

CALORIES: 392 TOTAL FAT: 28g PROTEIN: 23g CARBOHYDRATES: 11g FIBER: 3g NET CARBS: 8g

CONVERSIONS

COMMON CONVERSIONS
1 gallon = 4 quarts = 8 pints = 16 cups = 128 fluid ounces = 3.8 liters
1 quart = 2 pints = 4 cups = 32 ounces = .95 liter
1 pint = 2 cups = 16 ounces = 480 ml
1 cup = 8 ounces = 240 ml
¼ cup = 4 tablespoons = 12 teaspoons = 2 ounces = 60 ml

TEMPERATURE CONVERSIONS	
Fahrenheit (°F)	Celsius (°C)
200°F	95°C
225°F	110°C
250°F	120°C
275°F	135°C
300°F	150°C
325°F	165°C
350°F	175°C
375°F	190°C
400°F	200°C
425°F	220°C
450°F	230°C
475°F	245°C

VOLUME CONVERSIONS		
U.S.	U.S. equivalent	Metric
1 tablespoon (3 teaspoons)	½ fluid ounce	15 milliliters
¼ cup	2 fluid ounces	60 milliliters
⅓ cup	3 fluid ounces	80 milliliters
½ cup	4 fluid ounces	120 milliliters
⅔ cup	5 fluid ounces	160 milliliters
¾ cup	6 fluid ounces	180 milliliters
1 cup	8 fluid ounces	240 milliliters
2 cups	16 fluid ounces	480 milliliters

WEIGHT CONVERSIONS	
U.S.	Metric
½ ounce	15 grams
1 ounce	30 grams
2 ounces	60 grams
¼ pound	115 grams
⅓ pound	150 grams
½ pound	225 grams
¾ pound	340 grams
1 pound	450 grams

RECIPE INDEX

ABOUT THE AUTHOR

Pamela Ellgen is a food blogger and cookbook author of *Sheet Pan Paleo, Cast Iron Paleo, The Microbiome Cookbook, Soup & Comfort*, and *Modern Family Table*. She also writes on fitness and nutrition, and her work has appeared on LIVESTRONG, Spinning.com, and the *Huffington Post*. When she's not in the kitchen, Pamela enjoys surfing, practicing yoga, and playing with her kids. She lives in California with her husband and two children.